EHAD with GOD

Biblical Healing Through Sanctification and Transformation In Christ

EHAD with GOD

Biblical Healing Through Sanctification and Transformation In Christ

Shaynah Neshama, PhD

This book is a work of nonfiction. Names and places have been changed for the protection of privacy.

Scripture is taken from the HOLY BIBLE, NEW INTERNATIONAL VERSION©.
Copyright©1973,1978,1984 by International Bible Society. Used by permission of Zondervan Publishing House. All rights reserved.
The "NIV" and "New International Version" trademarks are registered in the United States Patent and Trademark Office by the International Bible Society. Use of either trademark requires the permission of the International Bible Society
Printed in the United States of America
Paperback ISBN: 979-8-9921506-1-2

Dedicated to my beloved boys
Joseph, Rumen, Emmanuel, Daniel, and Elijah

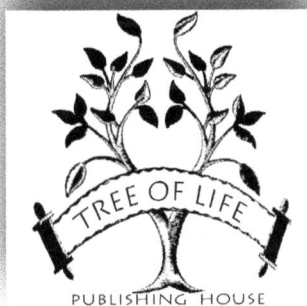

TABLE OF CONTENTS

Acknowledgments

God is my ghostwriter, editor, and distributor. I only had to submit in the wee morning hours when His voice would be the clearest. This is His book. I am the conduit, delivering His deep knowledge of the things unseen for the healing of many. All Eternal gratitude, honor, and praise belong to Him. Thank you, My God, Lord, and Savior, for the exhilarating ride on the wings of Your infinite wisdom, now available for the benefit of Your people.

Words cannot adequately express my gratitude to my family when I say, "Thank you." For the many hours when my mind would be following celestial navigation while performing mundane tasks around the house, without noticing your presence, I ask, please forgive me. For the many times when I would be emotionally unavailable to talk because my thoughts would be galaxies away, please forgive me. For the many missed opportunities to say, "I love you," please forgive me. Your love was the fuel that propelled me across the finish line. It will take an eternity to reciprocate your kindness. Thank you, my husband and boys.

To the saints in my life, my dearest friends in Christ, I say, "Thank you." You faithfully carried me on the wings of your prayers. Thank you, Ben and Margaret Ward, Roya and Nick Vetter, Jeannine and David Christian, Annette and Michael Feller, your friendship is immeasurable in earthly units. You all have been instrumental in what God is doing in my life. Thank you, Fred Harvey, a true saint, for recruiting me to work with you in the challenging but rewarding field of prison ministry. Your name is well-known in the Kingdom of God and makes the enemy tremble.

Thank you, Pastor Doug Brown. You made the deep things of God known to me, and your pastoral care for the brokenhearted a model to follow. Thank you, Vineyard Church in Claremont, California, for anointing me for service and sending me to the "four corners of the world" to teach and make disciples of all nations. Thank you, Pastor Doug Lindley, for your immeasurable support on every step of my ministry to God's people in crisis. Thank you, First Baptist Church and Hoover Valley Mission in Burnet, Texas, for entrusting the most vulnerable in my care. May Hoover Valley be known as the Valley of Healing.

Special recognition to the giant support of Chaplain Mark Cartwright and the entire staff at Ellen Halbert prison unit in Burnet, Texas. Your commitment to serving the downtrodden is my model to follow. As I witness your tireless dedication and service, my spirit tunes to God's Spirit for the plea of suffering. The *EHAD with GOD* methodology for healing from trauma was developed while working under your guidance. Thank you.

Rabbi Stuart Dauermann, you are my spiritual mentor in Messianic Judaism and the voice of Christ in my life. Your teaching on the doctrine of EHAD is legendary, and I am now passing it on to a new generation of believers. Thank you to all my friends from Ahavat Zion Synagogue, California, for your love and prayers.

To Sofia Baptist Church, Bulgaria, I say, "Thank you" for nurturing me at the well of living waters to grow into a mighty oak of righteousness. I am eternally grateful to Fikiya Milanova and her beautiful family. God used you in amazing ways to minister to me. Thank you for your servant's heart.

Thank you to the designers Raymond Zeal Fillingim from Faith Academy, Marble Falls, Texas, and Kralen Dickerson, Kingsland, Texas, for your unique art and craftsmanship, which capture the essence of my work.

Last but not least, to all my friends from California, Texas, Kentucky, Bulgaria, Prague, the Czech Republic, and Russia, who have touched my life with the blessing of Christ, I say, "Thank you," for being the light of Christ in a world of pain and suffering. Because of your love, I love too. May our Good Lord bless you tenfold for the kindness you have shown me.

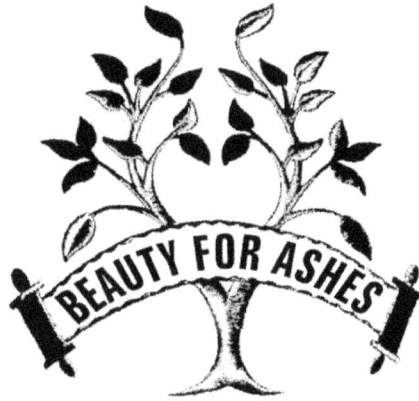

SESSION ONE

INTRODUCTION

EHAD with GOD is a biblical methodology for healing from traumatic events and spiritual oppression. It forms a healing alliance with God to bind up the brokenhearted, liberate the captives, and release the prisoners bound in spiritual darkness (Isaiah 61:1). Christ said, "I have come that you may have life, and have it abundantly" (John 10:10). The reality in the Church, however, is different—it is full of broken people, lacking abundance in life. The usual culprit is unresolved issues with anger, hatred, resentment, and unforgiveness harbored toward "those who trespassed against us" (Matthew 6:12). These are practices of the flesh that constitute a "foothold" (Ephesians 4:27) for Satan to steal, kill, and destroy. They are strongholds of darkness that serve as open doors, giving legal permission to the enemy to oppress, deceive, and harass. It is a spiritual captivity, causing a serious impediment to spiritual growth.

The *EHAD with GOD* approach identifies these areas of spiritual oppression and guides the believers to redeem them through the cross, cutting off the enemy's access to their lives. For this reason, *EHAD with GOD* is structured as a one-on-one biblical prayer counseling guide for healing from trauma and can be used in the privacy of a believer's home. It incorporates the spiritual tools and spiritual disciplines commonly utilized in Christian counseling and pastoral care practices. The Holy Sacraments of the Church of confession, repentance, and forgiveness are the bedrock on which this approach is built.

EHAD is a Hebrew word (אחד) and stands for being ONE with God. It reflects the sole purpose of the biblical narrative to encounter God and know Him personally, evoke a deep love toward Him, and, ultimately, become united with Him for eternity (John 14:20; 17:23).

Trauma may vary in the circumstances it occurred, from early childhood trauma, physical, sexual, or mental abuse, war veteran, loss of a loved one, drug and alcohol addictions, victims of violence, crime, human trafficking, natural disaster, etc. Despite the different nature of these experiences, the healing from trauma follows the same road of divine healing. This is the road after which *EHAD with GOD* was designed.

EHAD with GOD adopts the term TRAUMA as an umbrella for all human experiences that thwart the believer from living life with Jesus to the fullest. From a spiritual perspective, the most minor and the most grievous traumatic events equally cause spiritual stagnation. In this book, the term TRAUMA refers to all traumatic human experiences, regardless of their scope, spectrum, or intensity.

EHAD with GOD guides believers to identify issues that prevent them from becoming ONE with Christ. Maturity in the faith requires purification and sanctification, leading to transformation in the image of Christ and freedom from spiritual oppression. The transition is marked by a change in the power that has dominion over the believer's life from "living in the flesh" to "living in the Spirit" (Romans 8:12-13). Freedom and healing from past wounds are side effects of a sanctified life.

The **goal** of *EHAD with GOD* is to help believers overcome brokenness and live life to the fullest (John 10:10). The main **objectives**:

1. Guide the believers to sanctify their lives (1 Thessalonians 5:23).

2. Lead the believers to grow from glory to glory in the image of Christ (2 Corinthians 3:18).

3. Make the believers perfect in agape love (1 John 4:20).

Instructions: The participants will learn, practice, heal, and mature through a 10-week curriculum. Each session is designed for one week of study, prayer, and reflection. Do not advance faster. Allow yourself time to absorb the teachings, apply the practical prayer guides, and reflect on your healing. Equip yourself with a Bible and a writing pad because many biblical references require access to their full text. Reflecting on your experience by recording your journey is highly recommended, as it has healing benefits.

The Narrow Road—The Road of EHAD with God

EHAD with GOD methodology adopts Jesus' instructions of walking on the narrow road and entering through the narrow gate into the Kingdom of God. Advancing through weekly sessions is like advancing on the narrow road toward eternity with Jesus.

> Enter through the narrow gate. For wide is the gate, and broad
> is the road that leads to destruction, and many enter through
> it. But small is the gate and narrow the road that leads to life,
> and only a few find it. (Matthew 7:13-14)

We are all on a journey toward eternity with God. It is not the actual time spent on journeying that is crucial to salvation, but the quality of that time. It is a matter of life and death that we work out our salvation with fear and trembling (Philippians 2:12). Take a moment to reflect on your life as a journey toward eternity with God. Jesus described only two options: The broad road that leads to destruction and the narrow road that leads to eternity with God. There is no middle road with "feeling good" compromises. On which road are you now? Are you advancing or stalled? Do roadblocks and hurdles beset your road? Are you in darkness? Are you lost? You are now encouraged to take an honest inventory of your spiritual life.

Question: How many years have you been in the faith? _____

Task: Rate the level of maturity in your Christian faith on a scale of one to ten, where one represents minimal maturity, and ten indicates complete maturity.

1   2   3   4   5   6   7   8   9   10
◯ ◯ ◯ ◯ ◯ ◯ ◯ ◯ ◯ ◯

Question: What criteria did you use to evaluate your maturity level? How have the years in the faith impacted your maturity in Christ? Are you satisfied?

_____
_____
_____
_____

> The Apostle Paul sets up an eternal criteria for maturity in the faith. In fact, though by this time you ought to be teachers, you need someone to teach you the elementary truths of God's Word all over again. You need milk, not solid food! Anyone who lives on milk, being still an infant, is not acquainted with the teaching about righteousness. But solid food is for the mature, who by constant use have trained themselves to distinguish good from evil. (Hebrews 5:12-14)

According to the Apostle Paul, maturity in faith is measured by the depth of understanding of the teaching of righteousness.

Question: How do you understand the teaching of righteousness? How are the virtues of righteousness attained in the believer's life?

_____
_____
_____
_____

Further, righteousness is an essential component of the Armor of God, as described in Ephesians 6:10-18. The believer must put on the breastplate of righteousness when dealing with the Devil's schemes.

Question: How do I put on the full Armor of God? How do I practically put on the breastplate of righteousness?

_____

_____

_____

_____

These and many other questions will be answered systematically, and biblical truths will be practically applied for the benefit of your freedom and healing. Record your answers in the space provided because, as we advance with each session, you will compare them later to your deepening understanding of the same spiritual matters.

Whatever your current situation is, do not despair. Hold on to Jesus' promises that He will never drive away those who choose to journey toward eternity with Him (John 6:37). Indeed, He would leave the ninety-nine and run after you to rescue you (Matthew 18:10-14; Luke 15:1-7). He has engraved you on the palms of His hands (Isaiah 49:16). He will never leave you nor forsake you (Hebrews 13:5b; Deuteronomy 31:6b). Come near to God, and He will come near to you (James 4:8).

The discussion that will follow teaches many foundational biblical doctrines. Before setting off to draw from the deep wells of biblical wisdom, it is prudent to pause for a moment of prayer, asking God for guidance.

Prayer

In faith, Lord Jesus, I ask that You shine Your light of understanding in my weary mind so my heart can comprehend the heavenly things that are beyond comprehension. I call upon Your Holy Spirit to teach me the truth of the Kingdom of God. I want to embrace Your ways so they become my ways. Jesus, guide my thoughts and feelings as I learn to step up on the narrow road toward eternity with You. Walk with me, Jesus, till the end and, along the way, turn my mourning into dancing (Psalms 30:11). I trade my ashes for Your beauty (Isaiah 61:3). I choose EHAD—to be one with you. Amen!

Unresolved trauma or relational conflicts are major obstacles on the narrow road. It is a significant impediment to spiritual growth in Christ. Emotional wounds, if not treated, can fester and cause many long-term mental health conditions, like suicidal ideation, attempted suicide, severe distress, anxiety, depression, substance use disorder, panic attacks, increased risk of promiscuous behavior, etc. These symptomatic behaviors are often rooted in deeply seeded spiritual conditions that manifest as physical ailments. When the principles of the narrow road are applied, the spiritual conditions are healed, and, in many cases, the physical ailments are also relieved.

On the narrow road, the pain from any traumatic event, insult, or offense is healed because the spiritual laws that govern the road ordain healing. They are divine tools for living life to the fullest under the circumstances of our fallen humanity. Each session's weekly readings, prompts, and assignments will direct your journey, with the end goal of propelling you through the narrow gate to eternity with Christ Jesus. On the narrow road, you will be guided to remove everything in your life that is incompatible with the Kingdom of God. You are encouraged to commit to a daily discipline of prayer and study so that the righteous attributes of Christ become your righteous attributes. You will be transformed into His likeness. The process of becoming more like Jesus is the process of sanctification; it is also the process of healing from traumatic events or offenses. A sanctified life is a spiritually mature life. John the Baptist said,

He must become greater; I must become less. (John 3:30)

The more Jesus in life, the less destructive are the powers of this world that wreak havoc on the soul. There are obstacles and roadblocks, floods, and storms that make the journey harder, sometimes to a degree that may deter you from pursuing your goal of becoming more like Jesus, thus thwarting your healing and maturity in the faith. To counteract these difficulties, the believer must commit to the foundational spiritual discipline of prayer.

EHAD (אחד)—Biblical Framework for Prayer Counseling

This therapeutic approach adopts the framework of EHAD as an overarching philosophy for healing from traumatic events. It is our Global Positioning System (GPS) on the narrow road. It is our blueprint for good health and living life to the fullest (John 10:10). The doctrine of EHAD is rooted in the sole purpose of the biblical narrative to encounter God and to know Him personally, to evoke a deep love toward Him with the ultimate purpose to become more like Him and be united with Him for eternity. Thus, the Hebrew word EHAD (אחד) means "to become ONE" or "to be united" with God. Adam and Eve became ONE (אחד) flesh upon their union.

> For this reason, a man will leave his father and mother and be united to his wife, and they will become ONE[1] [אחד] flesh. (Genesis 2:24)

Upon giving the Ten Commandments, God is identified as being EHAD (אחד). Moses charged the Israelites,

> Hear, O Israel! The LORD our God, The LORD is ONE [אחד]. (Deuteronomy 6:4)

Jesus explains to His disciples the essence of EHAD [אחד].

> I and the Father are ONE [אחד]. (John 10:30)

And again.

> On that day, you will realize that I am in my Father, and you are in me, and I am in you. (John 14:20)

In the garden of Gethsemane, Jesus prayed for the disciples,

> Holy Father, protect them by the power of your name—the name you gave me—so that they may be ONE [אחד] as we are ONE [אחד]. (John 17:11)

> I have given them the glory that you gave me, that they may be ONE [אחד] as we are ONE [אחד]. (John 17:22)

---

[1] The word ONE is capitalized to emphasize the meaning applied in the discussion

In the parable of the sower (Matthew 13), Jesus speaks of four kinds of seeds that represent four kinds of people. They all heard the gospel, the good news of salvation, but only one quarter will "produce a crop—a hundred, sixty or thirty times what was sown"(Matthew 13:9). Bearing fruit is a requirement for belonging to the kingdom of God. Only believers who abide in Jesus can bear fruit. Jesus spoke of himself as the vine and the believers as the branches (John 15). If believers remain in him, they will bear much fruit. Apart from him, however, one can do nothing. If anyone doesn't abide in Jesus, they are like a branch that is thrown away and withers; such branches are picked up, thrown into the fire, and burned (John 15:5,6). Abiding in Jesus is becoming EHAD with him.

> Abide in Me, and I in you. As the branch cannot bear fruit of
> itself, unless it abides in the vine, neither can you, unless you
> abide in Me. (John 15:3b,4 NKJV)

Apostle Paul considers his life achievements as garbage. Instead, he desires to "gain Christ and be found in him"[to be one with him, (NLT)] (Philippians 3:8). Apostle John calls for no compromise when seeking oneness with Christ.

> We must be in him [to be אחד with Him] who is true. (1 John 5:21).

The author of the letter to the Hebrews further explains.

> Both the one who makes men holy and those who are made
> holy are of the same family. (Hebrews 2:11)

The NKJV and the Hebrew version of the Jerusalem Bible translate "the same family" as "they are all of ONE" (אחד). Becoming ONE (אחד) with God is the condition for entering the Kingdom of God. One must become compatible with God's holiness and purity to enter the Kingdom of God. In His sermon on the Mount, Jesus proclaimed,

> Blessed are the pure in heart, for they will see God. (Matthew
> 5:8)

The same requirement for purity, as a condition for oneness with God, is echoed in the letter to the Hebrews.

Without holiness, no one will see God. (Hebrews 12:14)

The prerequisite for becoming ONE (אחד) with Jesus is to become more like Jesus. The healing from trauma and freedom from spiritual oppression are hinged on this condition. This healing approach is designed as an action plan for achieving a Christ-like life. Our end goal is to become EHAD (אחד) with Christ. Each session will take you on a journey to this end. You will, indeed, experience Jesus' promises to become EHAD (אחד) with Him. EHAD (אחד) with Christ is a transformation into His image. When achieved, this transformation brings healing from any trauma.

The Holy Sacraments of the Church

The principles of EHAD are built on the daily practice of confession, repentance, forgiveness, Scripture study, prayer, and Eucharist for renewal through the presence of the Holy Spirit. These are essential parts of the holy sacraments and constitute the priestly duties of the Church. Within the Catholic tradition, most of them can only be applied by an ordained priest. The evangelical practice allows, in addition to a pastor, any mature clergy or layman to administer these priestly duties, which align with the pastoral care and pastoral counseling practices of the Church. The biblical understanding of Jesus as our high priest (Hebrews 4:14-16) gives believers the right to approach God's throne of grace with confidence and enter His presence without fear, seeking confession, repentance, and forgiveness through prayer and worship. This is the process of **self-deliverance** from spiritual oppression. The teachings and the guided prayers throughout each session are designed with this purpose. They can be applied in the privacy of a believer's "inner room" or "prayer closet" (Matthew 6:6), as well as in small groups and ministerial practice.

Self—Deliverance From Spiritual Oppression

Deliverance is only effective in the framework of a long-term commitment to the daily practice of the above-stated spiritual disciplines: Confession, repentance, forgiveness, Eucharist, Scripture, and prayer for healing and renewal through the presence of the Holy Spirit. Jesus explains what happens in the spiritual realm if we omit to do so.

> "When an evil spirit comes out of a man, it goes through arid places seeking rest and does not find it. Then it says, 'I will return to the house I left.' When it arrives, it finds the house unoccupied, swept clean, and put in order. Then it goes and takes with it seven other spirits more wicked than itself, and they go in and live there. And the final condition of that man is worse than the first." (Matthew 12:43-45)

There is no vacuum in the spiritual realm. There is no "gray area" where one can retreat to a little corner, undisturbed by spiritual forces in the spiritual realm. There is God, and there is the Devil. Jesus explained:

> He who is not with me is against me, and he who does not gather with me scatters. (Matthew 12:30)

The Apostle Paul teaches that this world is governed by the ruler of the kingdom of the air (Satan), who is the spirit, working in those who are disobedient (Ephesians 2:2b).

Question: What or who occupies my "house?" Identify beliefs, goals, activities, desires, individuals, and things that drive your life.

_____
_____
_____
_____

Any identified areas incompatible with the Kingdom of God are the enemy's territory. A believer must learn to distinguish between holy and profane. God is present in the first, and the Devil is present in the second. The believer's body is God's temple. The Apostle Paul makes this clear:

Do you not know that your body is a temple of the Holy Spirit, who is in you, whom you have received from God? (1 Corinthians 6:19)

The Spirit of the living God must dwell in continuity in the believer's "house." Certain behaviors, thoughts, and actions can defile the "house" and cause the Holy Spirit to depart from it. Prophet Ezekiel records one of the most somber events in human history: God's departure from the Temple.

Then, the glory of the LORD departed from over the threshold of the temple. (Ezekiel 10:18a)

In ancient times, God's presence departed because the priests had defiled the temple with their abominable practices. In this age of the Church, engaging in carnal practices has the same effect. The believer must have a clear understanding that the manner in which we conduct our lives on earth determines our eternal destination—heaven or hell.

First, the believer's "house" must be occupied by the Spirit of the living God, or else, who takes residence? As Jesus taught in Matthew 12:43-45, an unoccupied "house" is taken over by the evil forces in the spiritual realm. The daily practice of the above-listed spiritual disciplines fills our "house" with the presence of God's Holy Spirit. Everything else is from the Devil.

Second, the continuous practice of sin serves as a "foothold"(Ephesians 4:27) for Satan and his minions to steal, kill, and destroy (John 10:10). Sinful behaviors are open doors that give access to the enemy to oppress, deceive, and harass a believer. They give the enemy legal permission for entry. Only repentance from those sinful practices and genuine turning away from them can evict any unwanted occupier and close the doors. Healing from traumatic events requires that all open doors be identified and closed immediately through a genuine confession and repentance. This is the process of **self-deliverance**. The subject will be discussed and practically applied in depth in the ongoing sessions.

The matter of your healing is a spiritual transaction between you and God. As you call upon Him, your awareness of His presence will exponentially increase. Approaching God requires an honest examination, a genuine confession, and wholehearted repentance. You are to stand before Christ, Your Lord, God, and Savior, in the privacy of your "inner room."

> There is one God and one mediator between God and men, the man Christ Jesus. (1 Timothy 2:5)

Jesus is our high priest, and we can approach Him with the task of confession and repentance.

> Therefore, since we have a great high priest who has gone through the heavens, Jesus the Son of God, let us hold firmly to the faith we profess. For we do not have a high priest who is unable to empathize with our weaknesses, but we have one who has been tempted in every way, just as we are—yet was without sin. Let us then approach the throne of grace with confidence, so that we may receive mercy and find grace to help us in our time of need. (Hebrews 4:14-16)

Come to Jesus for confession, repentance, and forgiveness of sin. If you confide in a friend, a priest, or a pastor for confession and repentance, you are encouraged to do so. Seeking help and guidance from these individuals is a personal matter between you and God. These individuals must be mature Christians, bearing Christ's likeness. A confidant can be any member of the body of Christ, not only a paid minister. The principle of the priesthood of all believers gives us the right to this practice.

> Therefore, confess your sins to each other and pray for each other so that you may be healed. The prayer of a righteous man [woman] is powerful and effective. (James 5:16)

EHAD PRAYER FOR HEALING

1. **IDENTIFY** practices of the flesh (behavior, character traits, or weakness) incompatible with the Kingdom of God. For example, anger is a practice of the flesh that must be rejected, crucified, and cleansed from. An extensive list of the practices of the flesh is compiled on pages 20-21.

2. **CONFESS** and repent from the sinful practice of anger.

3. **CRUCIFY/PUT TO DEATH** anger, nailing it on the cross of Jesus.

4. **WASH IN THE BLOOD**. Claim the cleansing power of the blood of Jesus, spilled on the cross, to wash pure everything that has been defiled by the practice of anger.

5. **FILL UP WITH THE HOLY SPIRIT** instead of anger.

Life according to the flesh is death; life according to the Spirit is eternal life. The believer must, by the power of the Spirit, put to death the misdeeds of the body (Romans 8:12-13). Those who belong to Christ Jesus must crucify the flesh with its sinful passions and desires (Galatians 5:24).

There are two practical ways to crucify/put to death the flesh:

1. For the first option, you need a simple wooden cross, a nail, and a hammer. Write the practice of the flesh (anger) on a small piece of paper. Fold it so its content remains hidden—this is a private matter between you and Jesus. Nail the folded sheet of paper to the cross, saying the sample prayers, page 14.

2. Imaginatively, see yourself crucifying the practice of the flesh in the same manner described above, seeing yourself driving those nails through the condemned practice. Use the sample prayers, page 14.

Each subsequent session is designed to accomplish the tasks outlined above through three distinct components: Biblical instructions, a prayer guide, and personal reflection prompts. These steps ensure that the knowledge learned is a knowledge applied with the end goal of healing from trauma and maturing in the faith—becoming EHAD with Jesus.

EHAD PRAYERS

Step 1. The Mercy of God

The first prayer in your journey of transformation is for God's mercy. This is, without doubt, the most important task you can ever undertake to position yourself eternally with God. Be encouraged and strengthened. Help is on the way! Our God is merciful. He desires mercy, not punishment or death (Hosea 6:6). He pardons sin and forgives the transgression. He delights in showing mercy (Micah 7:18). His mercy is available to anyone who accepts it. God's mercy triumphs over judgment (James 2:13). A significant impediment to the acceptance of God's mercy is pride. You must humble yourself and plead for mercy and pardon. Approach God and accept His mercy for healing from trauma.

Over two thousand years ago, Jesus proclaimed the year of the Lord's favor (Isaiah 61:2). It has spiritual benefits for all humanity. Seek God with all your heart, soul, and strength while He can still be found. Today is the day of the Lord's favor for you. You will know the moment of your healing when you will indeed say:

> I will praise you, Oh LORD ... I will trust and not be afraid. The LORD, the LORD, is my strength and my song; He has become my salvation. (Isaiah 12:1,2)

Prayer for Mercy

Father, brokenhearted, I come before You in the name of Your Son, Jesus Christ. I bow before You and proclaim You as my Lord, God, and Savior. To You, I come in my distress because there is no one like You. There is no one who can understand; there is no one who has compassion and shows mercy. In Your great compassion, turn Your fierce anger into a life-giving river. I come to You, God, the Giver of Life, the Fountain of Living Water, and I ask that You deal with me according to Your steadfast love. Oh Lord, have mercy on me.

I am tired of wandering around. I am thirsty and hungry deep within. I have gone my ways, and I have done my things. I have taken a lot but have remained empty. Nothing fills me with good measure to satisfy the longing in my heart. Have mercy on me, the sinner, for I have become senseless and idle towards Your holy presence. Forgive my ignorance, Father. I deserve nothing but the stern discipline of Your righteous hand. Oh Lord, have mercy on me.

I pray now that Your hand extends to me for blessing instead of destruction. Break the iron shell around my heart; turn up Your holy fire in me and melt the ice inside. Make me soft and sensible again. Remove the heart of stone within and give me a heart after your own heart. Remove the veil of darkness from me. Let Your presence penetrate the core of my being as water penetrates the arid land of a desert. Soak me in Your goodness and revive in me the joy of Your salvation. Do this, Lord God, not because I deserve it but because of Your great Name. Oh Lord, have mercy on me. I pray in the name of my Lord, God, and Savior, Jesus Christ. Amen!

An earnest plea for mercy sets you on the path of restoration. The next step requires your sincere, wholehearted confession and repentance. It calls for an honest examination of heart and mind.

Step 2. Examine Yourself

There is no communion with God, no coming closer to Him, without first being cleansed from the impurity of sin. We must examine ourselves before we partake in the Holy Communion and eat of the bread and drink of the cup in remembrance of Jesus (1 Corinthians 11:28-30). Why do we have to examine ourselves? According to the Scripture, failure to examine ourselves properly leads to weakness, sickness, and even death. However, if we judge ourselves, we would not come under judgment (1 Corinthians 11:31).

What are we to examine or, as the Apostle Paul said, to judge? We must examine every area of life—from our relationships to our attitudes toward God and others. We must judge every character trait—from thoughts and feelings to flaws and habits. A thorough examination is essential to the healing from traumatic events. In addition to examining attitudes and behavior, there is still another test, an ultimate test, the Apostle Paul urges us to take.

> Examine yourselves to see whether you are in the faith; test yourselves. Do you not realize that Christ Jesus is in you— unless, of course, you fail the test? (2 Corinthians 13:5)

The Apostle Paul warns bluntly,

> If anyone does not have the Spirit of Christ, he does not belong to Christ. (Romans 8:9b)

Those to whom Paul writes are all believers in Christ. They have been saved and have experienced the redemptive power of the cross. Paul's call for examination is for you today. What test, you may ask, would authenticate the presence of the Spirit of Christ within? The passing mark is the presence of the fruit of the Spirit:

> Love, joy, peace, patience, kindness, goodness, faithfulness, gentleness and self-control. (Galatians 5:22)

Examination weighs up the believers' character against the presence of the fruit of the Spirit. Everything we build through our efforts is marked by unrest. Everything God builds is distinguishable by His seal of peace. Achievements and riches leave us unfulfilled, thus steering our appetites for more and more of the same, creating an upward spiral of unquenchable desires built on our wants and the effort to satisfy them. The spiral, though, never seems high or strong enough. It demands constant fueling for building consequent levels, leaving us dissatisfied and setting us up for new pursuits for fulfillment.

This is a sad displacement of the only true source that can satisfy the soul's deep longing. As a result, the soul remains malnourished, which ultimately leads to spiritual illness and an inability to commune with God. True satisfaction comes from the peace Jesus imparts in the heart of the believer.

How do I find rest and peace? Crucify the areas of unrest on the cross. By dying to the old nature in Jesus, we also rise in Him, transformed and renewed into His likeness. Death on the cross demolishes the power of the areas of unrest over the believers' lives. Resurrection transforms these areas into the likeness of Christ. It is a gain for eternity!

Before we take something to the cross, however, we have to identify it. This is the process of self-examination. As with everything else, even our examination is ineffective without God's involvement. God brings the secret thoughts and attitudes of our hearts out of darkness and into His light. The Lord tests the heart and is pleased with integrity (1 Chronicles 29:17a). The deep motives of our thoughts, desires, and intentions are distorted even for us. Knowing this, King David cried out to God,

> Search me, Oh God, and know my heart; test me and know my
> anxious thoughts. (Psalms 139:23)

King David's prayer should also be our prayer, inviting the Holy Spirit to participate in this crucial step of the healing process.

Prayer For The Guidance of The Holy Spirit

Spirit of the Living God, come and descend on me. Come and fill me up. I invite You to minister to me. I desire Your presence. Fill up my heart with Your holy fire. Shine on me Your holy light. Search me and bring to mind areas of my life that have not yet come into conformity with the Kingdom of God. Make me aware of the flaws of my character that are still holding me a prisoner to sin. Examine the aches of my heart and make me see the roots that cause them. I surrender all to You, Lord Jesus. Search me and know me. Give me the strength to bring to Your cross the sinful practices of my old self. I don't want any part of me left to slavery; I want the life of freedom I have in You, Lord Jesus. I pray in the name of my Lord, God, and Savior, Jesus Christ. Amen!

Step 3. Identify Areas that Have Dominion over Your Life

Identify the problem behaviors and character traits inconsistent with the Kingdom of God. Described below is a practical way to examine areas of unrest in a believer's life. You can implement it in the privacy of your inner room (Matthew 6:6). Take time to do what Apostle Paul suggests, and examine yourself (1 Corinthians 11:28-30; 2 Corinthians 13:5).

Read prayerfully through the list of behaviors, flaws, weaknesses, and character traits listed in **Table 1.** Rate them on a scale from one to ten according to the gravity of oppression over your life. The list is only suggestive. Add any other areas that are relevant to your life.

Look through the list you have compiled. Read out loud each area you have identified. These are the strongholds of evil over your life. These are the hooks with which evil holds you captive to sin. They have enslaved you. You have come to accept them as part of your identity. Shake off the lies! You are not what the enslaving power of sin makes you appear to be. You are a beloved child of God and an heir of the heavenly Kingdom. Do not allow anything else but royal blood to run through your veins and transform you into the King's likeness.

Arrange the problematic areas based on their severity over your life. Prioritize them according to your need to free yourself from their bondage. Bring them to God in prayer, one at a time. Be aware that by doing so, you are entering into a battlefield in the spiritual realm. It is a battle for your life. A broken and penitent heart that voices a prayer for repentance and forgiveness is the most potent weapon the Lord has given you to tear down strongholds of evil in your life.

> For though we live in the world, we do not wage war as
> the world does. The weapons we fight with are not the
> weapons of the world. On the contrary, they have divine
> power to demolish strongholds. (2 Corinthians 10:3-4)

Come, bow humbly before the Lord God, your Maker. Confess your sins and repent of your ways. Let the Holy Spirit minister to you as you open your heart for divine healing. Allow this to take as long as necessary for your confession to be wholehearted. Tears are okay. Jesus does not despise tears; He cries with and for us.

Blessed are those who mourn, for they will be comforted. (Matthew 5:3)

Note: Remember to accept God's forgiveness upon your confession if you pray alone. If you pray with a confidant, that person must pronounce forgiveness over you, and you must accept it. An earnest prayer of confession and repentance brings forgiveness immediately (John 20:23).

Prayer for Confession and Repentance of Sin

Lord God, I have sinned against You. Father, I come in the name of Jesus to ask forgiveness for my sin of _____. I have deliberately trespassed Your Law. It is a grievous sin I have committed against You, Father. I was foolish and ignorant. I confess that I have allowed my mind to be blinded by the darkness of this world and my heart hardened by its evil ways and inclinations. I repent from giving ear to these lies and believing in the deception. Forgive me, Jesus, for straying away from Your true teachings. Pardon me, Oh Lord! Bring me back into the fold of Your presence. Blot out the grievous sin I have committed. I can no longer carry this heavy load. Brokenhearted, I humbly come to Your cross and seek Your pardon. Forgive me, Lord Jesus. I pray in the name of my Lord, God, and Savior, Jesus Christ. Amen!

Table 1: Rate each practice of the flesh according to its power over you, with 1 being the lowest and 10 the highest, negatively impacting your life.

Practices of the Flesh					SCALE					
Anger/Rage	1	2	3	4	5	6	7	8	9	10
Bitterness	1	2	3	4	5	6	7	8	9	10
Hatred/Contempt	1	2	3	4	5	6	7	8	9	10
Envy	1	2	3	4	5	6	7	8	9	10
Shame	1	2	3	4	5	6	7	8	9	10
Vengeance	1	2	3	4	5	6	7	8	9	10
Unforgiveness	1	2	3	4	5	6	7	8	9	10
Self-condemnation	1	2	3	4	5	6	7	8	9	10
Pride	1	2	3	4	5	6	7	8	9	10
Control	1	2	3	4	5	6	7	8	9	10
Laziness	1	2	3	4	5	6	7	8	9	10
Foul Speech	1	2	3	4	5	6	7	8	9	10
Judgmental Attitude	1	2	3	4	5	6	7	8	9	10
Gossip	1	2	3	4	5	6	7	8	9	10
Disrespect to Parents	1	2	3	4	5	6	7	8	9	10
Gluttony	1	2	3	4	5	6	7	8	9	10
Alcohol Abuse	1	2	3	4	5	6	7	8	9	10
Drug Abuse	1	2	3	4	5	6	7	8	9	10
Pornography	1	2	3	4	5	6	7	8	9	10
Sexual Perversions	1	2	3	4	5	6	7	8	9	10
Lust	1	2	3	4	5	6	7	8	9	10

Adultery	1	2	3	4	5	6	7	8	9	10
Fornication	1	2	3	4	5	6	7	8	9	10
Fear	1	2	3	4	5	6	7	8	9	10
Lying Tongue	1	2	3	4	5	6	7	8	9	10
Deception	1	2	3	4	5	6	7	8	9	10
Stealing	1	2	3	4	5	6	7	8	9	10
Fame	1	2	3	4	5	6	7	8	9	10
Love for Money	1	2	3	4	5	6	7	8	9	10
Mistreating Others	1	2	3	4	5	6	7	8	9	10
Arrogance	1	2	3	4	5	6	7	8	9	10
Spiritual Slumber	1	2	3	4	5	6	7	8	9	10
Unbelief	1	2	3	4	5	6	7	8	9	10
Falsehood/Hipocracy	1	2	3	4	5	6	7	8	9	10
Lack of Trust in God	1	2	3	4	5	6	7	8	9	10
Disobedience/Rebelion	1	2	3	4	5	6	7	8	9	10
Impatience	1	2	3	4	5	6	7	8	9	10
Guilt	1	2	3	4	5	6	7	8	9	10
Murder	1	2	3	4	5	6	7	8	9	10
Occult Practices	1	2	3	4	5	6	7	8	9	10
Coveting	1	2	3	4	5	6	7	8	9	10
Jealousy	1	2	3	4	5	6	7	8	9	10
Greed	1	2	3	4	5	6	7	8	9	10
Selfishness	1	2	3	4	5	6	7	8	9	10
	1	2	3	4	5	6	7	8	9	10

Step 4. Crucify Practices of the Flesh at the Cross

Bring the practices of the flesh you just identified to the cross of Jesus. They must be condemned to death on the cross. This is a spiritual transaction in which, out of obedience to Jesus, you must deny yourself, take up your cross daily, and follow Him (Luke 9:23). Begin with the most urgent issue that has the strongest hold over your life. Afterward, deal with less challenging problems at a self-set pace.

There are two practical ways to magnify the spiritual significance of this crucial step. The application of either one produces the desired results.

For the first option, you need a simple wooden cross, a nail, and a hammer. Write the practice of the flesh on a small piece of paper. Fold it so its content remains hidden—this is a private matter between you and Jesus. Nail the folded sheet to the cross, saying the sample prayer below.

For the second option, imaginatively, see yourself crucifying the sins in the same manner described above, driving those nails through the condemned practice. Use the words of the sample prayer below.

Prayer for Crucifying a Specific Sin

Jesus, broken and needy, I come to You and confess my inability to conquer the sin of _____ in my life. I now renounce this practice of the flesh and desire to turn away from it. I say "NO" to it. I don't want this sin in my life. I hate it because it is evil. I don't want anything to stand between You and me, Jesus. Forgive me.

Now, I consciously exercise my free will and reject the slavery to this sin. I take the sin that torments my life and nail it on Your cross. This burden of sin does not belong to my heart. It belongs to Your cross, for You died for all of my sins, and this particular sin. I desire to die to this part of my sinful, carnal nature. I reject it. I condemn it to death on your cross. I declare this sin dead and turn away from it in Jesus' name. Amen!

Bring to the cross each problem area you have identified and deal with it in the same manner: Confessing, repenting, renouncing, and nailing it on the cross. Repeat the act of repentance for every sin you identified. Do not deal with all problems in one prayer session. Allow the Holy Spirit to minister to you without the pressure of time.

Step 5. Forgive Others

Just as you have asked the Father to forgive your sins, you must also extend forgiveness to those who have sinned against you. Rid yourself of all the pain you have kept inside by forgiving those who caused it. It is heaven's way. It is a spiritual law. Rendering forgiveness to those who have hurt you has the power to release you from the bondage of pain. Without forgiveness for others, God can't forgive you.

> If you forgive men when they sin against you, your heavenly Father will also forgive you. But if you do not forgive men their sins, your Father will not forgive your sins. (Matthew 6:14-15)

This principle is embedded in the Lord's prayer as well,

> Forgive our debts, as we have forgiven our debtors. (Matthew 6:12)

You must find the strength to forgive people who have wounded and grieved you. You may find yourself overwhelmed with negative emotions, unable to forgive. Yes, it isn't easy to forgive a perpetrator of an offense. Emotions are raging. Feelings override reason. You want to do what is right, but cannot follow through. Here is some practical advice to remember:

GO WITH THE MOTION, NOT WITH THE EMOTION

Be sincere in your prayer request. Pray in all earnest. A prayer from the depths of the heart is heard loudly on high.

Prayer for the Forgiveness of Others

Father who art in heaven, I honor You by obeying Your commandment to forgive those who have trespassed against me. I come to You wounded by _____. I need Your grace, Father, to find strength to forgive. Empower me to release my heart from the bondage of unforgiveness towards _____. I choose to forgive _____ from the depths of my heart. Father, don't count anything against _____ for the offense he/she has committed against me. I pray in the name of my Lord, God, and Savior, Jesus Christ. Amen!

Step 6. Release Bitterness, Resentment, Hatred, and Anger

As discussed earlier, harboring resentment, bitterness, animosity, hatred, and anger is self-destructive. These are sinful practices that cause unredemptive emotional pain. You must forgive those who caused you to react sinfully. Now is the moment to ask the Holy Spirit to search your heart and examine it for any roots of bitterness, anger, hatred, and resentment. The presence of the Holy Spirit brings to the surface feelings and emotions that have been long forgotten or buried.

Prayer Against Bitterness, Hatred, and Anger

Holy Spirit, I invite you to examine my heart for any traces of bitterness, resentment, hatred, and anger. Search me and bring every hidden thought and emotion that is an offense before You. Make me aware of the hidden roots of bitterness, resentment, hatred, and anger I may harbor toward some individuals. Bring them to my mind so I can recognize and renounce them. I forgive my offenders. Guide me through this process until these sinful practices no longer have power and dominion over my life. I pray in the name of my Lord, God, and Savior, Jesus Christ. Amen!

As you invite the Holy Spirit to minister to you, be aware of any thoughts, memories, or emotions that may suddenly flood you. These memories may come with a mental picture of an event that dates back to early childhood. The experience is often accompanied by Scripture verses, passages, or stories that speak in a revelatory manner about that specific event. God's ways of communication are awesome!

When, under the guidance of the Holy Spirit, you identify roots of bitterness, hatred, animosity, and anger, you must repent, renounce, and bring them to death on the cross. By doing so, you are freeing yourself from their enslaving power over your life. Upon your confession and repentance, according to the law of sowing and reaping, you will no longer reap the bad fruit of these practices because you have destroyed their root through death on the cross.

Step 7. Claim the Cleansing Power of the Blood of Jesus

Everything that sinful practices have defiled must be cleansed. Only the blood of Jesus, shed on the cross, can cleanse from sin.

Prayer for Cleansing

Lord Jesus, I claim the cleansing power of Your blood, spilled on the cross, to wash me pure from the defilement of my sins. Wash my mind and purify my thoughts. Wash my heart and purify its attitudes. Wash my entire body, from head to toe, and make me whiter than snow, purer than gold, and shinier than the sun. Cleanse me, for I desire to approach You blameless, pure in mind, body, soul, and spirit. Thank You, Jesus, for Your obedience to accept the suffering on the cross that now provides cleansing from my sin. I pray in the name of my Lord, God, and Savior, Jesus Christ. Amen!

Step 8. Deeper Cleansing of Mind and Heart

There is a need for a deeper cleansing from events and practices that serve as a huge open portal for the evil forces. Especially dangerous are any occult practices, drug and alcohol abuse, and sexual perversions. Their roots are buried so deep that we might not even be aware they exist. Ask the Lord to reveal these to you and let Him remove them from within your soul.

Prayer for Deeper Cleansing

Lord Jesus, I call forth Your sword of truth to cleave deep through my mind and heart. Anything within me that doesn't belong to Your Kingdom, please say a word and remove it; touch me and destroy it. Put the sharpened ax at the root of any planting the enemy has sown in me and cut it down. Clear my mind, Lord! Remove anything that has taken root and suffocates the growth of the true seed of Your Kingdom.

Likewise, Lord, clear my heart from lies and deceptions that have found fertile ground to grow. Remove, clear, cut down, and pluck out all the wrong attitudes and structures that belong to my old, evil practices of flesh. Establish Your truth in me. Thank You, Lord Jesus, for Your faithfulness to leave the ninety-nine (Matthew 18:12) and run after me to deliver me from my self-destructive ways of life. Thank you for returning me to the narrow road toward eternity with You. I believe, Lord, that the power of Your Word is sufficient to accomplish this. Speak Your goodness over me and continue Your refinement of my life until my old nature of flesh is completely transformed into Your likeness. I pray in the name of my Lord, God, and Savior, Jesus Christ. Amen!

Step 9. Call upon the Sanctifying Presence of the Holy Spirit

Cleansing from the defilement of sin is vital for obtaining spiritual and emotional health. Cleansing is an act of "emptying" yourselves from all that is yours. However, this is only half of the way towards sanctification. Once cleansed, we must be filled with the Holy Spirit. The Spirit's presence heals pain, sanctifies, and restores to righteousness. We are called to offer our bodies, cleansed and holy, as a dwelling of the Holy Spirit.

> If a man cleanses himself ..., he will be an instrument for noble purposes, made holy, useful to the Master, and prepared to do any good work. (2 Timothy 2:21)

Prayer for Sanctifying with the Holy Spirit

Spirit of the living God, come gently upon me. Holy Spirit, fill me up with Your sanctifying presence. Heal the brokenness inside. Restore to me the righteousness and the goodness as it was designed from the beginning of time. Gladden my soul with Your presence. Penetrate deep into my heart and my mind. Breathe on me Your breath of life. Make Your dwelling within me. Anoint me for service.

Teach me the Way of Holiness. Guide my walk in the way of the Kingdom of God. Equip me with strength from above to resist the temptations of the evil one, the world, and my flesh. Holy Spirit, set me apart. I desire to be holy because You, my God, are holy. Impart in me Your goodness, Your love, and Your peace. May Your righteousness be my righteousness, Your goodness be my goodness, and Your wisdom be my wisdom. May the life I live in this body be the life I have in You. May I no longer live, but You, my Lord Jesus, live through me. Thank You, my Lord, my God, and my Savior. I pray in the name of Jesus Christ. Amen!

Step 10. Declare Forgiveness and Blessings

It is done! You just did what Jesus said we would do:

> I tell you the truth, anyone who has faith in me will do what I
> have been doing. (John 14:12)

Jesus broke the strongholds of darkness over people's lives. In faith, you also broke the strongholds of darkness over your life and set yourself free, just as Jesus said we were to do. And now, based on your confession, repentance, and willingness to grow in the image of Christ, you are forgiven! You are absolved of your sins. In the name of Jesus, you are declared free from the bondage of sin. You are free from the enslaving power of unredemptive pain and heartache. You are cleansed and pure, spotless, clothed in white, sealed for all the good work the Lord God has accomplished in you. Now, read the triple priestly blessing and accept it for your life:

The LORD bless you and keep you; the LORD make his face shine upon you and be gracious to you; the LORD turn his face towards you and give you peace. (Numbers 6:24)

If you have chosen to go through this process with a confidant, ask that person to pronounce the above blessing over you. You must believe that it is done! You took the scriptural steps to heal the pain from trauma. You made a giant step to sanctify your life. The healing of your heart has begun because you are on your way to being transformed in the image of Christ.

Attention! You must also know that before your state of heart gets better, it will get worse. Don't be discouraged! Be informed! There is a turning point at which the old structures of flesh are replaced with new structures bearing the likeness of Christ Jesus. This point is marked by unrest, uneasiness, heaviness, and pain. One feels more burdened after taking the practices of the flesh to the cross than before this step. The reason for this condition is embedded in the process of dying to one's self and rising anew in Christ. Physical death is not pleasant or easy; neither is spiritual death any different, especially death on the cross.

Don't be discouraged if you experience the same thoughts and emotions that tormented you for so long. You are very likely to continue experiencing heartache, but the pain is bound to lose its power with each affliction. The degree of suffering may vary, depending on your stance against it. You must continue claiming the one most important thing you have done: You renounced your old ways, thinking structures, attitudes, bitterness, resentment, anger, or whatever other areas of your life were problematic. You placed them on the cross and reckoned them as dead. They are dead indeed! It is a spiritual law. The changes in the spiritual realm have already occurred. Even though you may not be aware of them yet, you must accept the healing by faith. It is only a matter of time until your awareness of the transformation increases. The physical changes lag behind the spiritual reality. For a permanently evident change, you must commit to a daily discipline of prayer for sanctification and transformation. You must claim daily the power of the cross for your healing. You must live up to what you have already attained (Philippians 3:14). And what you have attained is the healing of your heart by faith in the Word. You achieved what the Scripture promised—freedom from the enslaving power of sin. You took the road of healing in faith. You must accept the fact of your healing by faith. Do not be deceived by feelings or thoughts of failure! Remember, the heart is deceitful above all things and beyond cure (Jeremiah 17:9).

Don't be enslaved again by old emotions, feelings, and behaviors, for the Scripture tells us not to put confidence in the flesh (Philippians 3:3). Instead, hold on to the Word of God because it is eternal, the same yesterday, today, and tomorrow. By doing so, you will experience the blessing of being the righteous who live by faith (Habakkuk 2:4).

One Week—Walking by Faith, Not by Sight

You must pray the EHAD prayers daily for one week. It is not that the "work on the cross" is not done. Indeed, upon your free will, you have crucified the old structures and thus have demolished their stronghold over your life. In the spiritual realm, this is now a reality. Yet, you are encouraged to practice these steps (page 13) for a week so that your mind can agree with your spirit, recognizing that your victory is indeed a reality on earth as it is in heaven. One week of consistent practice of the above steps has shown to be effective in overcoming the old habits of the flesh. The old structures of thinking and the old inclinations of yielding to emotional pain are slow to conform to the new spiritual reality. Stay the course for one week, and soon, you will stand in the holy assembly, testifying to your newfound freedom. In about one week, what Jesus has done in your heart in the heavenly realm will become a reality on earth.

Don't be surprised at what is happening! Be prepared instead and knowledgeable to respond adequately. Don't allow yourself to think, even for a moment, that what you have done failed to deliver healing. Demonstrate unwavering faith. Because you have crucified your old self, your old self is indeed dead now. What you might be experiencing again are rumblings of old patterns of thinking and feelings that call for instant gratification. These old ways wish to survive and contend against their demise. They tend to have lives of their own for a while because they are products of the old flesh. They continue to surface even though the source of their origin has been demolished. The old practices lack an underlying structure to support life within them anymore. They are indeed dead. With time, the urges subside and fade into history.

Remember! The enemy, the Devil, will throw at you anything to discourage you. When you find yourself enticed by old thoughts, emotions, and attitudes of the heart, it is in your will and power to stop them. They are indeed dead. Show discipline, resist the Devil, and he will flee from you (James 4:7). Pray the Armor of God prayer (page 317). Soon, you will find your heart pain-free. This is the point at which your mind agrees with your heart that the oppressive practices of the old flesh are gone.

Death on the cross is slow and painful. Resurrection afterward is not immediate. It took Jesus three days and three nights in the heart of the earth (Matthew 12:40). How long will it take for your sinful nature of flesh to die? How long will it take for the newly resurrected life in Jesus to replace the old structures of flesh with God-filled righteousness and holiness? It all depends on how firmly you stand in faith to resist the forces of darkness and claim your new self formed in the image of Jesus Christ.

You must continue to renounce daily any residues of your old nature of flesh and haul them to the cross. Crucify them! Cleanse yourself in the blood of Jesus and be filled with the healing presence of the Holy Spirit (page 13). Believe that what you have done on earth has also been done in heaven. The power of your prayers has stirred into motion a set of events in the spiritual realm to complete this process. Your prayer, spoken in faith on earth, was heard in heaven and has become a reality in your life.

The prayer pattern above must become your daily spiritual discipline. It assures your victory over the old ways of life. It affirms your continuous walk on the narrow road. Your misery will turn into bliss. By committing to the prayer of sanctification and transformation in the image of Christ, we commit to "always carry around in our body the death of Jesus, so that the life of Jesus may also be revealed in our body." (2 Corinthians 4:10-11).

Why the Pain? Why the Suffering?

The biblical view on healing integrates physical and spiritual health into the understanding of human wellbeing. A close study of Jeremiah 29:11 reveals a deeper understanding of God's perspective on our welfare.

"For I know the plans I have for you," declares the LORD,

"plans to prosper you and not to harm you, plans to give you

hope and a future." (Jeremiah 29:11)

This verse is often engraved on items as delicate as exceptional art pieces and as mundane as T-shirts and bumper stickers. It is often spoken as a promise of hope and vision for the future to grieving or greatly discouraged people. For the happy and the prosperous, this verse has no weight. For the brokenhearted, the verse may sound very personal and yet distant. Personal, because God's words sound intimate, spoken at an eye level communication contact, and distant because the future is always uncertain for those living in pain when happiness, health, and prosperity seem unattainable.

The plans, however, that the Prophet Jeremiah talks about are not the plans God has for just a particular individual, even for the brokenhearted. This is God's Grand Plan forged back at the beginning of time in the Garden of Eden. This is God's Plan for humanity's deliverance from the consequences of the Fall. Because of its grand purpose, this Grand Plan benefits all individuals, the entire human race. Healing from traumatic events and offenses is embedded in God's Grand Plan.

God's Grand Plan

God's Grand Plan was spoken into motion in the Garden of Eden. Eden was the perfect place, created for a thriving human life with no illness, pain, or death. Nature was also perfect, with no earthquakes, hurricanes, fires, floods, or tornadoes. The perfection of life in Eden had God's divine seal of approval, "It was very good" (Genesis 1:31). Everything was perfect until, through deception, the Devil manipulated Adam and Eve to disobey God's only commandment—not to eat from the Tree of Knowledge of Good and Evil. As a result, death came into humanity (1) and nature (2) alike, just as God had said it would.

(1) For dust you are, and to dust you will return. (Genesis 3:19)

(2) The creation itself will be liberated from its bondage to decay. (Romans 8:23)

Since the Fall, humanity and nature have been going into an entropy mode, from disintegration and gradual decline into chaos, towards ultimate annihilation. God's Grand Plan is a divinely designed intervention to stop the advancement of this destructive course and save the human race from the curse of death. Sole faith in Jesus reverses the curse, turning it into a life-giving blessing. God's Grand plan for the redemption of humanity and nature began at the time of the Fall. God said:

> And I will put an enmity between you and the woman, and between your offspring and hers; he will crush your head, and you will strike his heel. (Genesis 3:15)

The serpent's offspring is Satan; the woman's offspring is Jesus. The enmity between both—one aims at the demise of humankind, the other aims at its salvation. God's Grand Plan spoke of victory for the human race over the destructive work of Satan. His plan was set in motion in ancient times, and it is now continuously unfolding before our eyes. But even more, Jesus was chosen as the Redeemer before the creation of the world to execute God's Grand Plan (1 Peter 1:20). Astonishingly, in the grand scheme of schemes, even we, who profess faith in Jesus were chosen in Him before the creation of the world to be holy and blameless in His sight (Ephesians 1:4). It is breathtaking to grasp that before God spoke the world into being, His Grand Plan was already set in place. On the sixth day, even before God created humanity, He foreknew everyone who would say "YES" to His call for salvation.

> For those God foreknew, he also predestined to be conformed
> to the image of his Son. (Romans 8:29a)

What a mystery! Yet, it is according to God's good pleasure to put this mystery into effect when the times reach their fulfillment, namely to bring all things in heaven and earth together under one head—Christ Jesus (Ephesians 1:10). Even though this fullness of time has now been revealed, as long as we are still on this side of eternity, God's divine providence will remain a mystery for us, the mere mortals.

Back to Jeremiah 29:11, the Hebrew word translated as "to prosper" (NIV) is "shalom" (שלום). Different Bible versions have translated this particular use of the word "shalom" (שלום) as "wellbeing," "welfare," or "peace" (NKJV). It is not accidental that the prophet used this exact word because the message it conveys is eternal. "Shalom," which means "peace" in Hebrew, is the indwelling of God's Holy Spirit. This is the same "shalom" (שלום) Jesus promised to the disciples and to all who would believe in Him.

> Peace [שלום] I leave with you; my peace [שלום] I give you.
> (John 14:27)

Jesus is the Prince of Peace (שלום) (Isaiah 9:6). Only through faith in Him can His peace become our peace. This peace surpasses all understanding and guards our hearts and minds in Christ Jesus (Philippians 4:7). Being armed with the gospel of peace (שלום) is a part of the full Armor of God, a must-have arsenal for spiritual warfare (Ephesians 6:15).

Jesus is the cornerstone of God's Grand Plan (Ephesians 2:20-22; Acts 4:11; Isaiah 28:16; Psalms 118:22). He defeated death and restored humanity's immortality. He also restored the glory with which humankind was created in God's image and likeness.

> But our citizenship is in heaven. And we eagerly await a Savior from there, the Lord Jesus Christ, who, by the power that enables him to bring everything under his control, will transform our lowly bodies so that they will be like his glorious body. (Philippians 3:20-21)

> And we, who with unveiled faces all reflect the Lord's glory, are being transformed into his likeness with ever-increasing glory, which comes from the Lord, who is the Spirit. (2 Corinthians 3:18)

Lord Jesus is also restoring Eden's glory. The book of Revelation describes a new heaven and a new earth.

> Then I saw a new heaven and a new earth, for the first heaven and the first earth had passed away, and there was no longer any sea. I saw the Holy City, the new Jerusalem, coming down out of heaven from God, prepared as a bride beautifully dressed for her husband. (Revelation 21:1-2)

For the believers with the Messiah's perspective, God's Grand Plan is the complete restoration of humankind and nature to their former glory in the Garden of Eden. This is the same glory God Himself imparted in us upon creation at the beginning of time (Genesis 2:7), which consequently was lost due to the Fall. Humankind regained its former glory through Christ crucified. On the cross, Jesus paid the penalty for the original sin. He crushed the ugly reality of death and restored the divine glory to us. We are propelled into eternity, becoming EHAD with God, just as it was in the Garden of Eden.

Consecration and Sanctification

In the Old Testament, God gave instructions to Moses on how the Israelites must prepare themselves before meeting with Him on Mount Sinai.

> And the Lord said to Moses, "Go to the people and consecrate them today and tomorrow. Have them wash their clothes and be ready by the third day, because on that day the Lord will come down on Mount Sinai in the sight of all the people. (Exodus 19:10,11)

Upon entering the Promised Land, Joshua gave similar instructions to the Israelites.

> Then, Joshua said to the people, "Consecrate yourselves, for tomorrow the Lord will do wonders among you." (Joshua 3:5)

King David consecrated himself before worshiping God.

> Then David got up from the ground. After he had washed, put on lotions, and changed his clothes, he went into the house of the Lord and worshiped. (2 Samuel 12:20)

Consecration in the Old Testament required washing with water and changing clothes, which signified bodily purity. Coupled with a penitent heart, this sets the person in the right standing with God. King David exemplified this attitude.

> My sacrifice, O God, is a broken spirit; a broken and contrite heart you, God, will not despise. (Psalms 51:17)

The Lord God states this spiritual law clearly.

> For this is what the high and exalted One says—he who lives forever, whose name is holy: "I live in a high and holy place, but also with the one who is contrite and lowly in spirit, to revive the spirit of the lowly and to revive the heart of the contrite. (Isaiah 57:15)

Physical cleanliness and a humble attitude of heart form a state of purity that was required before making a sacrifice on the altar for the remission of sin.

The Temple practices, based on Leviticus 20, required that before entering the Temple Mount, worshipers bathe in a specially designed for this purpose "mikvah" (ritual bath). Archeological excavations have found many of these baths around the southern wall. In the tunnels of the western wall, a large bath, Sanhedrin Mikvah, was discovered, just about 65 feet from the Western Wall. The Ophel Mikvah was most likely used by the Temple priests and was excavated not far from the southern wall.

> Consecrate yourselves and be holy, because I am the Lord
> your God. Keep my decrees and follow them. I am the Lord,
> who makes you holy. (Leviticus 20:7,8)

The text clearly indicates two distinct parts. The first part, the worshipers must undertake on their free volition and consecrate themselves. This is **consecration**. The second part, God makes the worshipers holy upon their consecration. This is **sanctification**. Without consecration, there is no sanctification. It is God who makes the believer holy! (Leviticus 20:8).

The *EHAD with GOD* approach embeds these two requirements. The EHAD prayer (page 13) leads the reader through the steps of consecration (steps 1-4). The believer must identify the practices of the flesh (step 1), confess, renounce, and repent from them (step 2), crucify them (step 3), and wash in the blood of Jesus (step 4). These steps appropriate the believer to enter the presence of God and to be sanctified, be made holy.

John the Baptist was a forerunner of Christ. He identified himself, by quoting Isaiah 40:3-8, as "the voice of one calling in the wilderness, 'Make straight the way for the Lord'" (John 1:23; Matthew 3:1-3). He called the people into repentance and baptism with water (Matthew 3:2-6). Just like in the Temple practice, John the Baptist consecrated the people, preparing them to meet God, Jesus Christ. Today, the believer must follow the same pattern of instructions before approaching God. We must adhere to Apostle Paul's call for consecration:

Therefore, come out from them and be separated, says the Lord. Touch no unclean thing, and I will receive you. (2 Corinthians 6:17)

Apostle Paul was quoting Isaiah 52:11, which outlines the path for consecration:

Depart, depart, go out from there! Touch no unclean thing!

Come out from it and be pure... (Isaiah 52:11)

God, through the voice of Apostle John in Revelation 18, reinforced the same message:

Then I heard another voice from heaven say: 'Come out of her, my people, so that you will not share in her sins, so that you will not receive any of her plagues.' (Revelation 18:5)

EHAD with GOD takes Apostle Paul's instructions seriously and calls the believers to be separated from worldly practices. Instead, we must put to death the old practices of the flesh and consecrate ourselves.

Put to death, therefore, whatever belongs to your earthly nature: sexual immorality, impurity, lust, evil desires, and greed, which is idolatry. Because of these, the wrath of God is coming. You used to walk in these ways, in the life you once lived. But now you must also rid yourselves of all such things as these: anger, rage, malice, slander, and filthy language from your lips. Do not lie to each other, since you have taken off your old self with its practices and have put on the new self, which is being renewed in knowledge in the image of its Creator. (Colossians 3:5-11)

"... put off your old self, which is being corrupted by its deceitful desires; to be made new in the attitude of your minds; and to put on the new self, created to be like God in

true righteousness and holiness. (Ephesians 4:22-24)

The Old Testament is a shadow of the things that transpired in the New Testament. As Apostle Paul says, "These are a shadow of the things that were to come; the reality, however, is found in Christ" (Colossians 2:17). The New Covenant is simultaneously a blood and love Covenant. Blood covenant, because the sacrifice on the cross satisfied the wrath of God and reconciled humanity with Him. It is a love covenant because it testified to God's divine agape love for all humanity, which made him sacrifice himself so we can have eternal life with him.

Today, the Cross brings a new dynamic as it comes to the consecration of the believers. While we should not neglect our physical state of cleanness, inner purity defines our pursuit. Confession and repentance, just like in the Old Testament, continue to be powerful spiritual tools for the demolition of strongholds of darkness over believers' lives. The power of the blood of Jesus spilled on the cross, however, has a new, distinctive function from that of the animals' blood required in the Temple practice: It is sufficient to atone and cleanse all humanity from all iniquity, once and for all. "Putting to death" the old self for the believer is the volitional act of crucifying the old nature with its corrupt practices on the cross of Jesus. This is step three from the EHAD PRAYER for healing approach on page 13. Once we cleanse our house (Matthew 12:43-45), we must keep it filled with the Spirit of the living God. Step five is an invitation to the Holy Spirit to indwell the believer. The EHAD PRAYER is our strongest weapon in the believer's arsenal of the armor of God.

Consecration is something we do prior to approaching God. **Sanctification** is from the Lord. Once we consecrate ourselves, He makes us holy by imparting His Spirit of Life, the Holy Spirit.

Salvation and Sanctification

God's Grand Plan is the redemption and the healing of humanity. Redemption is the personal experience of salvation, a defined moment in time and space when a confession of faith in Christ as the Messiah is made. On the other hand, healing is the lifelong experience of sanctification through which the believer sheds the old nature of self and, in the process, is endowed with the righteousness and holiness of Christ, leading to transformation in His image and ultimate glorification.

> And those he predestined, he also called; those he called, he also justified; those he justified, he also glorified. (Romans 8:30)

The process of **sanctification** is the biblical understanding of healing and freedom from spiritual oppression. Salvation and redemption, sanctification and healing, are the premises on which *EHAD with GOD* progresses throughout the healing process. It is a spiritual transaction in which personal free will, exercised in the physical realm, unfolds its power to actuate spiritual matters in the spiritual realm. Salvation resurrects the dead human spirit. Sanctification stops the corruption of the soul, transforming it into a Christ-like character. Healing from trauma is a process through which the believer progresses through sanctification and, in the process, becomes EHAD with Jesus. As Apostle Paul affirms,

> Therefore, if anyone is in Christ, he is a new creation: The old has gone, the new has come! (2 Corinthians 5:17)

The "new creation" may have the scars (like Jesus does) but not the pain. Isaiah describes the spiritual transaction that happened on the cross:

> But he was pierced for our transgressions, he was crushed for our iniquities; the punishment that brought us peace was on him, and by his wounds we are healed. (Isaiah 53:5)

EHAD is healing, and EHAD happens on the narrow road. Becoming EHAD with Jesus is the ultimate goal of this healing journey. As we keep moving on the narrow road, we shed off the old nature with its corrupt practices of the flesh, and we are mystically infused with Christ's divine nature. His righteousness becomes our righteousness, His wisdom, our wisdom; His joy, our joy, His peace, our peace. On the cross of Jesus, a splendid trade happens daily. As we lay down our old nature with its sinful practices and desires, Jesus Himself bestows on us a crown of beauty instead of ashes, the oil of gladness instead of mourning, and a garment of praise instead of a spirit of despair. We are called oaks of righteousness, a planting of the Lord for the display of his splendor (Isaiah 61:1-3).

Growing in the image of Christ is **sanctification**. It is not an optional destination for the believer; it is a command to be perfect because our heavenly Father is perfect (Matthew 5:48). The call to be perfect is not unattainable. It is a call to sanctify our lives. And this effort lasts to the end: We must run the race to get the crown (2 Timothy 4:7).

Salvation and **sanctification** are two sides of the same coin. While salvation by faith in Christ is a determined point in time, sanctification through Christ is a lifelong walk with Him on the narrow road toward eternity. Healing from the ruptures of a traumatic event is the process of sanctification. *EHAD with GOD* takes you on that transformative journey from pain to peace (שלום).

Prayer

Jesus, I desire your healing. Your sacrifice on the cross saved me, Your blood washed me pure. Now, sanctify me, Lord. Set me apart for eternity with You. I stand at Your cross, and I exchange my filthy rags for Your beauty. I submit to You. Slow me down, Lord. Sharpen my sight and quicken my mind. Give me a willing spirit. Grant me an undivided heart as I commit my mind, spirit, soul, and body to complete devotion to You. Cause me to absorb your teachings and make them my life-giving guide. I choose to become EHAD with you. I pray in the name of my Lord, God, and Savior, Jesus Christ. Amen!

EHAD with GOD

REFLECTION—Week One

Reflection 1: Give Him Five (5 minutes)—the daily practice of God's presence (see description on this page and 63 under "Deep calls to deep" section).

Reflection 2: Daily confession, repentance, and crucifying the practices of the flesh (see pages 13, 14 for instructions).

Reflection 3: Read Psalm 91 and respond to the question below.

Reflection 4: Initial Assessment—Physical and Spiritual Triage

Reflection 5: Evaluate four areas of your life as they stand today

Reflection 6: In The Quiet of My Kitchen

Reflection One—Instructions

1. Give Him Five (5 minutes). Set aside five (5) minutes daily, and find a place and time you will be least disturbed. Even though circumstances may not allow for peaceful seclusion, you can find solitude in your heart amidst crowded and brightly lit spaces. Close your eyes and invite the Spirit of the living God to take you to His land of promises. Leave the land of loneliness and be transported to the land of solitude. Choose solitude.

2. Pray the above prayer repeatedly (page 40) so that the mind and heart agree with your words spoken in faith.

3. Spend time talking and listening to Jesus. Learn to recognize His voice. Practice His presence. You will be amazed!

Task: Reflect on "Give Him Five" time with Jesus in prayer today.

_____

_____

_____

_____

Reflection Two—Instructions

Daily confession, repentance, and forgiveness before the Lord Jesus, our high priest. Crucify the practices of the flesh (see page 13 for instructions). Write your prayer that reflects your struggles with the old nature. Reflect on your experience.

Psalm 91

Read Psalm 91 and respond to the question below. The original "he/him" nouns are replaced with "I" and "you" nouns so that the message sounds much more personal.

I say

The one who dwells in the shelter of the Most High, will rest in the shadow of the Almighty. I will say to the LORD "You are my refuge and my fortress, my God in whom I trust!"

The Promise

Surely he will save you from the fowler's snare and from the deadly pestilence. He will cover you with his feathers, and under His wings you will find refuge. His faithfulness will be your shield and rampart. You will not fear the terror of night, nor the arrow that flies by day, the pestilence that stalks in the darkness, or calamity that destroys at noon, nor the plague that destroys at midday. A thousand may fall at your side, ten thousand at your right hand, but it will not come near you. You will only observe with your eyes and see the punishment of the wicked.

If you make the Most High your dwelling—even the LORD, who is my refuge—then no harm will befall you, no disaster will come near your tent. For he will command his angels concerning you to guard you in all your ways; they will lift you up in their hands, so that you will not strike your foot again a stone. You will tread upon the lion and the cobra; you will trample the great lion and the serpent.

The LORD says

"Because you love me," says the LORD, "I will rescue you. I will protect you, for you acknowledge my name. You will call upon me, and I will answer you."

"I will be with you in trouble. I will deliver you, and honor you."

"With long life will I satisfy you and show you my salvation."

The promises in Psalms 91 are God's promises for you. The Lord God desires one and only one thing in His relationship with you—your love for Him to reciprocate His love for you. "'Because you love me', says the Lord," I will do all the things listed under *The Promise*. Looking retrospectively at your life, do we see your love for God throughout the years past? Do you love God? The Scripture says a lot about the way He loves you.

> You see, at just the right time, when we were still powerless, Christ died for the ungodly. But God demonstrates his love for us in this: While we were still sinners, Christ died for us. (Romans 5:6,8)

God's ultimate expression of His love is when He, on His own free volition, took the punishment for our trespasses on Himself so we can go free. Yes, the Creator of the Universe went through pain, suffering, and death for the entire human race, including you. If you were the only human on earth, He would still die for you. You may feel unseen, abandoned, ignored, shoved away, insignificant, trampled over, spat on, etc., but these feelings are subjective because the Creator elevates you to the status of His child, an heir of His Kingdom. He sees you not in your broken state of heart but in your glorified state in heaven. He has not finished His work with you until His holiness and righteousness are imparted in you, becoming EHAD with you.

Task: On a scale from 1 to 10, where 1 represents "no love," and 10 signifies "through-the-roof love," how do you measure your love for God? Take a moment to reflect on your findings.

1   2   3   4   5   6   7   8   9   10

○ ○ ○ ○ ○ ○ ○ ○ ○ ○

Task: On a scale from 1 to 10, where 1 represents "no love," and 10 signifies "through-the-roof love," rate God's love for you?

1   2   3   4   5   6   7   8   9   10

○ ○ ○ ○ ○ ○ ○ ○ ○ ○

Question: How does my love for God compare to His love for me right now?

_____
_____
_____
_____
_____
_____
_____
_____
_____
_____
_____
_____
_____

In the beginning, God created humankind out of love. After the Fall, God devised a plan to restore us to our former glory because of His love. God stepped into human history, and out of love, He executed His Grand Plan. The Scripture is a love letter to humanity—a divinely inspired instruction manual with directions on choosing life under the fallen condition of a dead world. Because He loves you, He created this exact moment in space and time just for you and Him to come together in fellowship and heal. He loves you because He has known you before He created the foundations of this world (Ephesians 1:4). God desires that you tone down, tune-up, and soar high on wings like the eagles (Isaiah 40:31). Today, He desires to affirm His promises to you listed in Psalms 91, saying, "I will do all these things for you because you love me."

Prayer

Father God, I searched my heart, and I found it lacking in love for You. Compared to Your love for me, my love for You falls short. I admit, I cannot love You with the same measure You love me. I ask You, Lord, to grant me the ability to reciprocate Your love. Impart in me, O Lord, Your divine love so I can love You with the same capacity You love me. I pray for Your divine love to flood me. In Your name, Jesus, I pray.

Initial Assessment—Physical and Spiritual Triage

An effective treatment plan requires an initial assessment to determine the degree of harm an individual has suffered due to trauma or relational conflicts. Trauma has adverse effects on the physical, emotional, mental, and spiritual well-being of the individual. At an emergency room, people are subjected to a clinical triage. It is a process that prioritizes cases based on the severity of their injury/trauma to determine if they require immediate or not-so-immediate medical treatment. From a spiritual perspective, we will also apply spiritual triage to assess the severity of the harm the trauma has caused to the soul/spirit. Similarly, like at an emergency room, doctors prescribe medications and apply specific treatment protocols. In our approach, the medicine has a divine nature, and our protocol follows the spiritual law for healing described throughout the biblical narrative.

Note: If you are taking any prescribed medication, follow the protocol. God is sovereign, and His healing is not limited by the presence or absence of medication. Clinical and spiritual triage serve as initial markers to map the state of overall health before and after *EHAD with GOD* treatment option. It has been observed that many physical, medical, and mental health conditions have been related to spiritual oppression. During the course of this study, often, when the spirit is healed, the body and its functions are restored as well.

Clinical Triage (Appendix 1)

Task: List the major physical health issues identified during the initial assessment.

_____
_____
_____
_____
_____
_____
_____
_____
_____
_____
_____
_____
_____
_____

Spiritual Triage (Appendix 2)

Task: List the major spiritual health issues identified during the initial assessment.

_____
_____
_____
_____
_____
_____
_____
_____
_____
_____
_____
_____
_____

Well-Being Scale For Self-Evaluation

Date _____

Evaluate four areas of your life affected by traumatic events. Mark your responses with "X" to the question: "How am I doing today?"

HOW AM I DOING TODAY	GREAT	OKAY	BAD	REALLY BAD	MISERABLE
PHYSICALLY					
EMOTIONALLY					
SPIRITUALLY					
RELATIONALLY					

Physically—My overall health. How solid is my night's sleep? My appetite, chronic conditions, current diagnosis, and quality of everyday life

Emotionally—Volatility of feelings, ups and downs of emotions, bouts of anger, rage, depression, manias, panic attacks, hatred, etc

Spiritually—Relationship with Christ, ability to worship corporately, read the Bible, prayer time, assurance of salvation, sense of God's presence

Relationally—Quality of familial relationships and circles of friends

Task: Record the results of your self-evaluation. Discuss your findings.

_____
_____
_____
_____
_____
_____

Spiritual Baseline

The following two paragraphs[2] describe two opposite spiritual states of mind and heart. As you read, identify the description that matches your current spiritual state of heart and mind.

Loneliness! Don't we all know this dry place well? A place where sheer silence attends to our wounds and absolute emptiness binds our bleeding hearts. A frightening place where Pain meets Sorrow, and together, they bring forth Despair. A place where we are forced to retreat for healing, only to find that our wounds have festered. A place where Loneliness has nested itself deep in our souls, creating a chronically ill state of heart. How so many of us know this place well!

Solitude! How few of us know this place well? A place where sheer silence reigns in quiet contentment and absolute is the serenity, not the emptiness. A blissful place where Joy meets Delight, and together, they bring forth Peace. A wonderful place where the wilderness inside blooms and the dry land flourishes, where the floods of joy spring into fountains of gladness and the gladdened soul soars on wings like the eagles. How very few of us know this blessed place well!

Loneliness is the trauma-imprisoned life, while solitude symbolizes freedom from pain and despair. Moving from pain and misery to healing is the transformational journey of becoming EHAD with Christ. Healing from trauma and spiritual oppression is a process of alignment of the human body, soul, and spirit with God's initial divine design, which was ordained at the beginning of time (Ephesians 1:4). Do you desire to undergo this marvelous transformation? Do you desire to depart from misery and find peace? Do you desire to encounter and obtain Christ's beauty (Isaiah 61:3)? Then, choose the narrow road of EHAD, becoming ONE with God, being in complete unity with Him.

---

[2] Excerpt from *Turn My Loneliness Into Solitude*, Shaynah Neshama. 2007, Tree of Life Publishing House, p. 11

Prayer

In faith, Lord Jesus, I come before your throne of grace and ask that you guide me on this healing journey. Touch me and heal me. Speak words of healing over me. Send me a blessing of relief. Take the pain away. Heal my heart, restore my dignity, renew my mind, and strengthen my faith. I desire to become EHAD with You, Jesus. I reject my old, corrupt ways of life and choose to be like You. Transform me into Your likeness, I pray. Amen!

Question: Which state of heart describes your current life—loneliness or solitude? Tell your story of pain and suffering to Jesus.

_____
_____
_____
_____
_____
_____

In The Quiet of My Kitchen

The pain was excruciating. It traveled fast from under my fingernail through the arm, reaching the core of my being. It fueled up a cry within. It flamed out my senses. It burned in a single prayer thought: "Lord, where are you to heal me the way you healed the servant's ear that night in Gethsemane when Peter took a knife and cut it off?" In that split second, my soul reached out for the only source of relief it knew.

Disgusted with myself, I had to face the harsh reality. I was now to endure the discomfort of my injured finger for the next few weeks. As I was washing the streaming blood, I kept blaming myself for not being careful enough with that forked-shaped, double-edged kitchen knife. After an intense morning of science lecturing, I was too tired, hungry, and impatient. The pounding in my head warned me of a quickly dropping blood sugar level. The cramps in my stomach urged me to hurry up. The thought of a freshly made sandwich blurred the precision of my hand-eye coordination. The knife flew out of my hand, piercing the flesh deep under my fingernail. My effort to alleviate the hunger left me with much greater trouble to bear.

The misery grew as my mind projected the pain that I was to endure weeks ahead. Not all households in my country enjoyed the convenience of a washing machine. Neither did my family. Public laundry machines were nonexistent. Hand washing the clothes used the day before was an essential part of my daily chores. Hand washing with a deep wound under my fingernail meant repeated pain, pain, pain. It was too high a price to pay in exchange for silencing my hunger.

The rest of the day went fast. The daily tasks around the house took my attention away from the accident. Only the tight bandage on my finger was a bitter reminder of my self-inflicted wound.

I did not deal with my injured finger until bedtime when I had to change the bandage. At the edge of my bed, I took time to gather strength and face the consequences of the injury. I knew lifting the bandage would cause pain, so I was careful. Slowly, I began revealing the affected area. With my finger in full sight, I could not see the exact spot where the tip of the knife had entered. Bringing it closer to my eyes did not help either. Touching it brought further disbelief. There was no sign of any injury. There was no incision, no pain, and no scar.

Did it ever happen? Had the tip of the knife really pierced deep under the nail? I recalled the pain, the blood washing down the drain, and the numbness of my entire arm. The bloody bandage, still in my hand, was clear evidence that what had happened earlier in the day was an authentic experience.

For the next few moments, my mind struggled to reconcile the sight of my completely uninjured finger with the memories of the incident. When everything came into focus, my cry at that moment stood out: "Where are you, Jesus?" I had cried out then. "Here I am" was the answer.

"Here I am." "Here I am." The words echoed in my mind throughout the night. My Lord, Jesus, had stood next to me. He healed me the way he healed that servant in Gethsemane 2000 years ago, just as I had prayed. He restored my flesh the way He had restored his. The Creator of the Universe took time to stand beside me and heal me. He did not perform this miracle on a big stage. He did not seek a large audience or any applause. Instead, He manifested His glory in the quiet of my kitchen. He did it for me, only for me.

That night, the Lord spoke to me clearly. As I reflected on this experience, I wondered at the attention I was given for injuring my little finger. After all, it was not a life-threatening injury but a small wound that would have healed in a few weeks. Then, I understood. It was a much bigger miracle; it was my heart that the Lord had healed.

During the previous months, I had been struggling with overwhelming doubts. I questioned the truthfulness of the Bible. I listened unconvinced to the pastor's message, wondering if he believed what he preached. The doubts had grown deep in my heart, affecting my faith and relationship with the Lord. In the light of the small miracle of healing, I grew immensely in understanding. It was not the healing of my finger that was the core of this event. His love entered deep in, uprooted the doubts, and prepared my heart for His Word to be inscribed on. His presence, the Lord Jesus himself, healed my disbelief.

Task: Rate your confidence level in God's healing from trauma, where 1 represents low confidence and 10 represents the highest confidence.

1	2	3	4	5	6	7	8	9	10
○	○	○	○	○	○	○	○	○	○

Task: Record your thoughts and reflect on your faith in divine healing.

_____
_____
_____
_____

Human Nature in Psychotherapy

Secular and Scriptural Perspectives

Psychotherapy and counseling emerged as distinctive scientific disciplines at the beginning of the 20th century as a result of the development of a new paradigm for treating acute psychiatric disorders. The new approaches reached beyond the biological factor to include a person's cognition, behavior, emotions, and belief system. Initially known as "talk" therapy and primarily applied as an assessment tool, it soon evolved to a much more elaborate level, including complex therapeutic interventions and their secular applications.

The development of trauma therapy could be likened to a miniature pattern of the development of the field of individual therapy, replicating the known therapeutic approaches but in condensed, time and space-constrained forms. The therapeutic strategies for treating traumatic experiences can be classified into four groups: Biological/mental, cognitive-behavioral, emotional, and spiritual.

Secular and Christian counselors view the application of the above approaches differently because their views on human nature differ. Secular counseling embraces the view of human nature as a dichotomy: soul (cognition/emotion) and body (behavior) relationship. Christian counseling views human nature as a trichotomy: soul (cognition, emotion), body (behavior), and spirit relationship.

Contemporary secular psychotherapy embraces the dichotomous approach. It is based on the cultural determinism of Emile Durkheim (1858-1917), a system built on the Marxist belief of perfecting the masses (in mind and cognition) through a change in the environment. Historically, this approach had a more direct impact on social policy-making than on direct therapist/client interaction. It promotes lobbying for changes in social laws that will improve society. The rationale behind this approach calls for a change in a person by providing a better environment that will ultimately usher in the brotherhood of global humanity. By its definition, the dichotomous approach looks only at a two-dimensional soul/mind and body human structure.

Secular psychotherapy recognizes that a therapeutic change is achieved when the healing of memories, changes in habits, and relationships happen. Healing occurs when the therapist provides satisfying insights into how past life events caused psychological changes and contributed to an individual's problematic functioning. In behavior therapy, healing occurs when new, socially acceptable forms of behavior are introduced to override the old, flawed habits, exerting self-control, which should lead to changes in a person's general demeanor.

In contrast to secular psychotherapy, *EHAD with GOD* applies the trichotomous approach, which adds an additional dimension, that of the spirit, to the structure of human nature. The EHAD framework for trauma therapy, introduced earlier, is consistent with the Judeo-Christian tradition of understanding human nature as a trichotomy: body, mind/soul, and spirit. Treating personality dysfunctions and relational problems begins with addressing the state of health/illness of the human spirit. This framework looks at healing as a process that starts with the gradual redemption of the old nature by systematically submitting it to spiritual death. Death is not an end but a prerequisite for renewed life. Therapeutic interventions are tailored according to the doctrines of healing and recovery through sanctification and transformation in the image of Christ.

All religions have a forgiveness component in their belief structures, and they all practice forgiveness as a volitional, spiritual act of absolution of guilt. A person does not have to be religious to benefit from forgiving others. Forgiveness is universal. One can judge by the sheer mass of professional publications on forgiveness to see that secular counseling has recognized the benefit of forgiveness. Often, forgiveness is understood as "being sorry" or "being apologetic." It is a part of most contemporary therapeutic approaches woven throughout different therapeutic techniques.

Christians and non-Christians suffer from trauma afflictions alike. The despair, the pain, and the damage to the hearts besiege both believers and nonbelievers. Both groups seem equally susceptible to trauma.

While the trauma afflicts Christians and non-Christians alike, both groups differ drastically in their approach to healing. The reason for this difference lies in understanding the trauma's root problem and its treatment, respectively. Depending on the personal convictions of the counselors, the ill effects of trauma are seen as broadly as being part of the package of human existence and as narrowly as being spiritual, psychological, or social. This variety of opinions leads to a variety of approaches for treatment. Secular counseling builds treatment strategies to address the physical manifestations of the trauma. Depression, social anxiety, promiscuity, anger, rage, addictions, panic attacks, eating disorders, bipolar disorder, PTSD, and the like conditions are treated through a combination of medication and therapy. Therapy builds on cognition, emotions, behavior, and the many versions of their combination. The most recent therapeutic approaches applied to trauma treatment include the method of eye movement desensitization and reprocessing (EMDR), which targets the memory associated with the trauma by desensitizing it, e.g., making it less painful.

These approaches omit the state of health of the human spirit. Without addressing the spiritual aspects, suffering, pain, and despair remain just desensitized. The trauma is buried deep in the victim's subconscious and, from there, can be triggered by unexpected life events.

The *EHAD with GOD* methodology for healing from trauma is trichotomous. It looks at trauma as rooted in the brokenness of the God-human relationship. A large group of professional Christian counselors shares this understanding. Life in pain proceeds from alienation from God for those who are outside the Kingdom of God and from immaturity in growing in the image of Christ for those who are saved and already belong to the Kingdom of God.

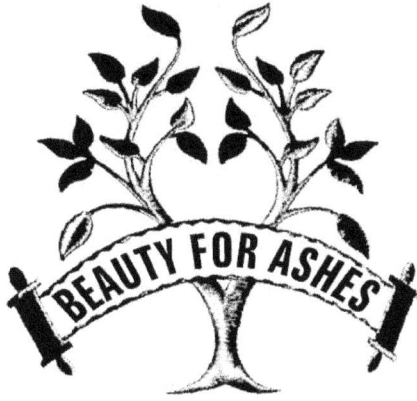

SESSION TWO

THE POWER OF THE SPOKEN WORD—PRAYER

The Mysteries of God

If there is a pattern that identifies God, it would be the consistency of God's mysteries. God says and does things that defy human reasoning. After all is said and done, no one will attribute the miracle to human effort but solely to the power of God. Two stories evidence this divine pattern.

In the **first story,** a Syrian general, Naaman (2 Kings 5), is suffering from leprosy. He had tried many doctors and shamans but found no cure. His Hebrew servant makes him aware of a prophet in Israel, Elisha, who can surely heal him. When Naaman arrives at Elisha's home, the prophet doesn't even meet him in person but sends his servant boy to give instructions for the cure. Naaman was told to dip himself seven times in the Jordan River. Naaman is furious, understandably angry for having traveled long distances to only be told to dip in the murky waters of Jordan. He fumed in indignation, ready to go back home. His servants, however, speak sense into him, and he agrees to follow through with the prophet's instructions. He dips himself seven times and is miraculously cured; "his flesh was restored and became clean like that of a young boy"(2 Kings 5:14). Naaman was angry because he thought that surely the prophet "would come out to me and stand and call on the name of the Lord his God, wave his hand over the spot and cure me of my leprosy" (2 Kings 5:11). His expectations were way off.

In the **second story,** Jesus makes a man born blind see again (John 9:1-12). His way of healing is astonishing. He spits on the ground, makes mud, and covers with it the eyes of the blind man, telling him to wash in the Pool of Siloam. The man went and washed, and came home seeing! Couldn't Jesus just touch the man's eyes, look up to heaven, say a prayer, and restore his sight on the spot? Why the mud? Or, are our expectations way off?

When our expectations don't match God's reality, we might become angry and rebellious, refusing to follow up with His instructions. We convince ourselves that the cure is too simple. Even more, because the cure is completely free of charge, how can it be of any value? Thus, we convince ourselves that such a simple way must not be the way for true healing. We would rather put our trust in expensive treatments offered by therapists and doctors with powerful titles and honorable degrees behind their names for the cure of our condition. Just like Naaman, when our expectations don't match God's reality, we might miss His healing. The *EHAD with GOD* approach is one such test of faith. Going through the motion of the five steps (page 13) is a simple gesture of faith, and when followed through in obedience, they result in a complete cure, freedom from emotional, physical, and spiritual oppression. The *EHAD with GOD* ministry (in church and prison) has a consistently high cure rate. When God is involved, the outcome is perfect because the approach is founded in God's irrevocable spiritual laws. Thus, don't reject God's Word and His laws, and God will not reject you. May the gift of faith from above be yours, delivering an eternal cure.

The Power of Faith in Prayer

The spoken word has enormous power in the spiritual realm. Prayer is the vehicle that propels the believer forward on the narrow road. Prayer is composed of words. In the spiritual realm, words have the power to build and to tear down; they have the power of life and death (Proverbs 18:21). God created the world by His Word. He spoke, and it all came to be!

> God said, "Let there be light," and there was light. (Genesis 1:3)

> By God's word, the heavens existed, and the earth was formed out of water and by water. (2 Peter 3:5b)

Jesus spoke His ministry into existence. He spoke and broke the chains of captivity from the minds of people. He commanded, and the evil spirits obeyed Him (Mark 1:27). He rebuked the storm, and it quieted (Luke 8:25). Jesus called out, "Lazarus, come out!" (John 11:43), and by the power of His Word, the process of decaying flesh was immediately reversed: A dead man resurrected before the astonished eyes of many. Jesus attested to the power of the words in prayer.

> The words I have spoken to you are spirit, and they are life. (John 6:63)

The spoken words affect our lives today as well. They have the power to bring death or life. Jesus said,

> For by your words you will be acquitted, and by your words you will be condemned. (Matthew 12:37)

When the Israelites suffered great thirst in the desert, God instructed Moses to speak to a rock at Kadesh,

> Speak to that rock before their eyes, and it will pour out its water. (Numbers 20:8)

Ezekiel was told to prophesy over dry bones, and they became alive.

> Then he said to me, "Prophesy to these bones and say to them, 'Dry bones, hear the word of the Lord! This is what

the Sovereign Lord says to these bones: I will make breath
enter you, and you will come to life. I will attach tendons to
you and make flesh come upon you and cover you with
skin; I will put breath in you, and you will come to life.
Then you will know that I am the Lord.'" (Ezekiel 37:1-28)

Jesus emphasized faith in action by insisting on the impossible: To tell a mountain to move.

Truly I tell you, if anyone says to this mountain, 'Go, throw
yourself into the sea,' and does not doubt in their heart but
believes that what they say will happen, it will be done for
them. (Mark 11:23)

Similarly, Jesus told His disciples,

I tell you the truth: whatever you bind on earth [in prayer] will
be bound in heaven, and whatever you loose on earth [in
prayer] will be loosed in heaven. (Matthew 18:18)

As recorded in the Book of Acts, the Apostles' lives were manifestations of their spoken words in faith. They preached, and, by the power of the spoken Word, in the name of Jesus, they healed and delivered many people from the bondage of evil.

To further affirm the power of the spoken word, consider what a blessing and a curse are. Each is a spoken word! Curses and blessings are embedded in the Law. They were enacted upon the giving of the Law; their unshakable authority remains today. The power of the spoken Word originates from the spiritual realm but affects the physical realm. Our own doing and speaking evoke forces that bring either blessings or curses to our lives. We reap what we have sown (Galatians 6:7).

The biblical patriarchs blessed their children. Abraham blessed Isaac (Genesis 27:28-29). Jacob blessed his twelve sons and prophesied their future (Genesis 49). The blessings are prayers that have prophetic power. Once spoken, the words of a prayer have a life of their own. The Bible records the fulfillment of the patriarchs' prayers over their offspring. Jacob's blessing over Judah (Genesis 49:8-10) included a prophecy that kings would come from Judah and that one King would eventually receive "the obedience of the nations." Judah's descendants later became the tribe from which King David came. Jesus Christ is a descendant of the tribe of Judah (Matthew 1:3). The blessing over Benjamin exhibits the same pattern. He was called a ravenous wolf set on devouring and plundering (Genesis 49:27). The tribe of Benjamin produced many military leaders in Israel, including King Saul and his son Jonathan, both of whom had strong warrior personalities (Judges 5:14; 20:16; 1 Chronicles 8:40; 2 Chronicles 14:8; 17:17).

Further, the high priests blessed the people with the Aaronic benediction, which is chanted in synagogues and prayed in churches worldwide, evoking God's name upon the worshipers for blessing and protection.

> The LORD spoke to Moses, saying, "Tell Aaron and his sons, 'This is how you are to bless the Israelites. Say to them, " 'The LORD bless you, and keep you; the LORD make his face to shine upon you, and be gracious to you: the LORD turn his face toward you, and give you peace." ' "So they will put my name on the Israelites, and I will bless them." (Numbers 6:22-27)

It is recorded that God's appointed ministers regularly spoke blessings over the people.

> The priests and the Levites stood to bless the people, and God heard them, for their prayer reached heaven, his holy dwelling place. (2 Chronicles 30:27)

The Apostle Paul tells us to bless God and bless His Holy Name. He starts his letter to the Ephesians with a blessing:

> Praise be to the God and Father of our Lord Jesus Christ, who has blessed us in the heavenly realms with every spiritual blessing in Christ. (Ephesians 1:3)

He also urges us.

Bless those who persecute you; bless and do not curse. (Romans 12:14)

Through the Prophet Zechariah, God reinforced to His people the validity of the curses embedded in the Law of Moses. In a vision of a flying scroll, the Lord warned the Israelites that the curses associated with the breaking of the Law were now going out over the whole land to accomplish everything according to what had been said (Zechariah 5:1-4). These curses continue to go out today, fulfilling God's Word in the lives of those who break His Law. We are also reminded that when the mouth of the Lord speaks, the words don't return to Him empty.

> As the rain and the snow come down from heaven, and do not return to it without watering the earth and making it bud and flourish, so that it yields seed for the sower and bread for the eater, so is my word that goes out from my mouth: It will not return to me empty, but will accomplish what I desire and achieve the purpose for which I sent it. (Isaiah 55:10-11)

The executing order in the spiritual realm is subjected to the power of the Word. Once spoken, it sets in motion forces within the spiritual realm that roll out and unfold until the spoken words come into existence in the physical realm and become a reality on earth as it is in heaven.

God's word is not chained! (2 Timothy 2:9)

Feelings or sensations do not necessarily accompany prayer. Sometimes they do. It is neither a rule nor an exception. Feelings should never override Scripture. We are being warned that the heart is deceitful above all things and beyond cure (Jeremiah 17:9).

The differences in our emotional response during prayer are embedded in how our physical and spiritual natures intersect with God's divine nature. For this reason, we have to be cautious about feelings and sensations coming from the heart, which can easily be mistaken for God's voice. God does use our feelings to speak to us, but so does the Evil One. In prayer, we test the spirits (1

John 4:1), and by testing them, we avoid the danger of falling into the traps of the enemy.

The ability to discern spirits and understand spiritual matters is a spiritual gift—the gift of discernment. It is developed by continually practicing prayer in the presence of the Holy Spirit. This gift is not restricted to theologically trained ministers but also to the brokenhearted.

Prayer should manifest our faith in action; it is not a display of feelings in idleness. We pray because we believe God hears. But even more, we pray because we believe God answers. Faith should not rely on feelings but instead on the unshakable assurance that God's irrevocable Word impacts the course of our lives immediately. Just like the prayers of the biblical patriarchs, our prayers also have the same prophetic power. We are encouraged to pray without ceasing (1 Thessalonians 5:16-18). Before ascension, Jesus assured His disciples,

> You may ask me for anything in my name, and I will do it.
>
> (John 14:14)

The process of healing from traumatic events is grounded in prayer. The practice of the spiritual discipline of prayer will take you through the stages of the healing process. You must begin this process with a correct attitude of the heart. Prayer brings you out from the static understanding of the roots of emotional pain to the dynamic action of eradicating it. Knowledge without prayer leads to foolishness; this is the way of the world. Likewise, an understanding of the root problem of emotional pain alone cannot alleviate it. Action is needed. Prayer is the combat vehicle for action against the oppression of emotional pain.

Prayer is also the "official" language of the Kingdom of God. Just as learning a new language requires time and effort, so does developing one's talking and listening abilities to God in prayer. These skills do not develop overnight, but once acquired, they remain for life. For every moment spent in prayer, God reciprocates with manifold blessings: The wisdom of the Almighty becomes your wisdom.

> I no longer call you servants, because a servant doesn't know
> his master's business. Instead, I have called you friends, for
> everything that I learned from my Father I have made known
> to you. (John 15:15)

This wonderful gift is ours when we practice the spiritual discipline of prayer daily; we actively establish God's will in our small corner of the world.

Subjectivism in Prayer

For many of you, the experience with prayer might be different, proving your effort worthless. You have prayed and prayed, but God has not answered. Shall we then presume that Jesus was untruthful, telling us to ask Him anything and He will do it (John 14:14)? No, our subjective perspective clouds our experience. We know very well what to ask, but do we know how to ask? Jesus tells us,

> But seek first his kingdom and his righteousness, and all these things
> will be given to you as well. (Matthew 6:33)

If we seek the Kingdom of God first, we are in full compliance with the first commandment.

> Love the LORD your God with all your heart and with all your
> soul and with all your strength. (Deuteronomy 6:5)

We also fulfill Jesus' command to abide in Him (John 15:4). Placing God first not only creates a right attitude of heart for presenting petitions before Him, but according to God's Word, it evokes God's promises of great blessings in our lives (Deuteronomy 28). There is an essential condition for an answered prayer:

> If you remain in me and my words remain in you, ask
> whatever you wish, and it will be given you. (John 15:7)

For an effective prayer life, we must abide in Christ, becoming EHAD with Him. The centrality of prayer is God and His kingdom. We pray because we want to see God and hear Him. We want to come closer to Him and experience His joy and love. In prayer, we approach God, and He approaches us. We know His will and participate in establishing it at that very moment and at the place He had positioned us. We participate in what He is doing in us, through us, and around us.

Deep Calls to Deep—Daily Practice of God's Presence

God is Spirit, and His worshipers must worship in spirit and truth. (John 4:24b)

Jesus set the appropriate conditions for approaching God: In spirit and truth. We must approach God in spirit because the realm of God is spiritual, and prayer is the language of communication within the spiritual realm. We enter into what King David describes as a "deep calls to deep" (Psalms 42:7) experience through prayer. This is a Spirit-to-spirit communication during which we reach the depth of God's heart and express the depths of our hearts in return. At this level, God reveals His wisdom to us by His Spirit because,

The Spirit searches all things, even the deep things of God. (1 Corinthians 2:10)

We must approach God in truth because this is God's very nature. God is truth, and we are to come to Him stripped of our old selves, which defile our minds with thoughts and our hearts with desires other than those of Him and His kingdom. To approach God in truth means to become transparent. Hiding and concealing thoughts, deeds, and attitudes work for people, not for God. The kind of transparency God wants us to achieve is transparency for both God and people alike: What people see in me is who I am without putting on a mask, trying to appear happy, good, intelligent, righteous, or knowledgeable. Jesus sternly warns that everyone who loves and practices falsehood is not allowed to enter through the gates of the city of God, the New Jerusalem (Revelation 22:15).

When we worship God in spirit and truth, we allow Him to work in us and transform us into His likeness. A life transformed in the likeness of Christ has a transparent quality because the heart transformed in the likeness of Christ becomes transparently pure.

The Spirit-to-spirit communication in "transparent truth" is the foundation of the God-person relationship. Spiritual growth requires that we seek this kind of depth in communication with our God; everything else is "chasing after the wind" (Ecclesiastes 1:14). At this depth, we can experience God as our heavenly Father because we have recognized Him as such and have approached Him as His children.

When the relationship of God-person reaches the depth of Spirit-to-spirit communication, we begin to truly experience and understand the depth of God's amazing love for us. It gently wraps around us, tenderly envelops us, and lovingly sings over us. One can grow "addicted" to the desire to experience God's love on this "deep calls to deep" level. This is the spiritual benefit of entering God's presence during prayer. The more one experiences it, the stronger one desires to have more of the same experience. This desire creates an inner longing that only heaven can fully satisfy. Until then, we are called to enter His presence daily in prayer. King David vividly described His own experience with God's presence as "deep calls to deep" (Psalms 42:7).

The morning prayer time of a believer has an unmatchable beauty. Once you evoke His name, He is beside you, ready to listen and commune with you. As you enter His presence, you become filled with anticipation and engulfed in His love. For a time, you are encouraged to remain there—without words of thanks, thoughts, praise, or petitions—simply taking in sincerely the delight of your Father's presence. In the beauty of that moment, you empty yourself of anything that is yours and allow your heavenly Father to fill you with everything that is His. This is the moment when, on your own volition, you strip yourself from the old nature with its corrupt desires and practices of the flesh and infuse yourself with the beauty of Christ. The Apostle Paul describes this spiritual act of divine exchange.

> I have been crucified with Christ, and I no longer live, but Christ lives in me. The life I now live in the body, I live by faith in the Son of God, who loved me and gave himself for me. (Galatians 2:20)

This trading is a pure spiritual barter in which your spirit and God's Spirit testify to the factual transaction. You literally experience heaven on earth. It is an exhilarating flight of the spirit that rises towards the height of the Father's Spirit, being absorbed in His divine presence. After such an assurance of His love, there is no way that one can agonize over trifling daily matters. You know in your spirit that, before a need arises, your heavenly Father has already seen it and has taken special care to provide for it. You may even wonder at the many times when you were not even aware of an approaching need because His divine provision had come down to you as a blessing, not as a need.

> He who searches our hearts knows the mind of the Spirit because the Spirit intercedes for the saints in accordance with God's will. (Romans 8:27)

The subject of the next section is how to achieve this depth of Spirit-to-spirit communication.

Power and Authority in Prayer

There is an epic display of the power of the Word in the world God created.

> Then God said, "Let us make man in our image, in our likeness, and let them rule [have dominion] over the fish in the sea and the birds of the air, over the livestock, over all the earth, and over all the creatures that move along the ground." God blessed them and said to them, "Be fruitful and increase

in number; fill the earth and subdue it. Rule over [have dominion over] the fish in the sea and the birds of the air and over every living creature that moves on the ground." (Genesis 1:26,28)

Without being created in God's image and likeness, there was no ruling (having dominion) over God's creation. God put Adam in charge of His creation. When the animals saw Adam, they also saw God. Similarly, when people later saw Adam's children, they knew they were his sons.

When Adam lived 130 years, he had a son in his own likeness,

in his own image; he named him Seth. (Genesis 5:3)

The Hebrew words for "image" and "likeness" in Genesis 5:3 and Genesis 1:26-27 express the same meaning, describing distinctive ancestral characteristics passed on from God to Adam and Adam to his sons. Since then, the image of God has been passed on from generation to generation to this day. When God created Adam, He breathed His breath of life in him, and he became a living being (Genesis 2:7). God imparted part of Himself into Adam. God did not place part of Himself in the rest of His creation; birds and animals don't have the divine impartation of God's breath of life. They don't have spirits. In the creation of humankind, the invisible and visible dimensions of God's creation came into existence—a full display of God's glory.

Bring my sons from afar and my daughters from the ends of the earth—everyone who is called by my name, whom I created for my glory, whom I formed and made. (Isaiah 43:7)

Angels are spirits, as are demons, who are considered fallen angels. They don't have bodies. For this reason, evil spirits tend to possess and oppress humans so they can experience human sensations and passions through the human senses. Since they are inherently evil, the behaviors they pursue are also evil. They defile and thus sever the ability for communion with God. In contrast, the impartation with the Holy Spirit has a sanctifying power that enables a Spirit-to-spirit relationship.

In the Garden of Eden, God gave one commandment to Adam and Eve with dire consequences if not obeyed: Not to eat from the tree of the knowledge of good and evil (Genesis 2:17). The serpent planted deception when questioning the truthfulness of God's warning: "You will not certainly die" (Genesis 3:4). Indeed, when Adam and Eve took the forbidden fruit, they saw that they didn't die. Didn't they? Being created after the image of God presupposes that, just like Him, humans are also three-in-one: Body, soul, and spirit. While it took Adam 930 years to die physically, his spirit died immediately at the time of the trespass. This condition of spiritual and physical decay is passed on to the entire human race as our ancestral heritage (Romans 5:12-19).

Only humankind intertwines in its nature, both the natural and the spiritual realms. The human spirit must be connected to God's Spirit for a healthy and fulfilled human existence. The human spirit must be alive to commune with the divine. After the Fall, the fullness of the image of God in humans was shattered; the likeness of God in humanity was marred because the human spirit died due to the trespass. Upon physical death, the body returns to the ground it came from, and the spirit returns to God who gave it (Ecclesiastes 12:7). Obedience to spiritual laws ensures that the human spirit remains alive and in communion with God.

Jesus, God Himself, came into human history to correct the course of human decay. He defeated death on the cross.

> Since the children have flesh and blood, he too shared in their humanity so that by his death he might destroy him who holds the power of death—that is, the devil—and free those who all their lives were held in slavery by their fear of death. (Hebrews 2:14-15)

Adam and Eve were created as immortals. They had access to the Tree of Life in the Garden of Eden and permission to freely eat its fruit. However, God took that privilege away upon their expulsion from the Garden of Eden. Adam and Eve were no longer immortals.

> And the LORD God said, "The man has now become like one of us, knowing good and evil. He must not be allowed to reach out his hand and take also from the tree of life and eat, and live forever." So the LORD God banished him from the Garden of Eden to work the ground from which he had been taken. After he drove the man out, he placed on the east side of the Garden of Eden cherubim and a flaming sword flashing back and forth to guard the way to the tree of life. (Genesis 3:21-24)

Reference to the Tree of Life in the Scripture only appears at the beginning in the book of Genesis and at the end in the book of Revelation. In Genesis, it provided immortality to Adam and Eve (Genesis 3:21). We can speculate that the gradual decrease in humanity's lifespan, recorded in the Bible, might have resulted from the banishment from accessing the Tree of Life. God later decreed:

> My Spirit will not contend with humans forever, for they are mortal; their days will be a hundred and twenty years. (Genesis 6:3)

"Living forever" (Genesis 3:23) without the corruption of sin is the divine design after which humanity was created in Eden. "Living forever" under the fallen condition was not allowed. Sin and immortality are not an option in the eternal divine design. This is the state of the Devil and the fallen angels. Restoration of humanity to the initial design had to satisfy the very spiritual laws God Himself spoke into existence.

First, God had to redeem us from the curse of death—this is **Salvation**. Second, God had to bring us into conformity with Himself—this is **Sanctification**. Only through these transformative conditions can humanity inhabit the New Jerusalem, where, under the new order of things, access to the Tree of Life is restored (Revelation 22:2).

There will be no more death, mourning, crying, or pain, for the old order of things has passed away. (Revelation 21:4)

The glory and the honor of the nations will be brought into to the New Jerusalem. Nothing unclean, and no one who does shameful things or tells lies will ever go into it. Only those whose names are written in the Lamb's book of life will enter the city. (Revelation 21:26,27)

Only those who wash their robes will have the right to the tree of life and will go through the gates into the New Jerusalem. (Revelation 22:14)

The New Jerusalem is the old Garden of Eden, where immortal humanity is EHAD with God.

Believers, born again by the Spirit of God, have regained the fullness of the "likeness" and the "image" of God. They were spiritually dead, but through faith in Jesus the Messiah, their immortality is restored because Jesus is not the God of the dead but the living (Mark 12:27). When people look at a believer, they should see Jesus. We represent Jesus. Jesus represented God. When the disciples saw Jesus, they saw the face of God. One day, the Apostle Philip asked Jesus,

"Lord, show us the Father, and that will be enough for us." Jesus answered: "Don't you know me, Philip, even after I have been among you such a long time? Anyone who has seen me has seen the Father. How can you say, 'Show us the Father'? Don't you believe that I am in the Father and that the Father is in me? The words I say to you are not just my own. Rather, it is the Father, living in me, who is doing his work. Believe me when I say that I am in the Father and the Father is in me, or at least believe on the evidence of the works themselves." (John 14:8-11)

The imprint of God's image on the believer is not only physical but also spiritual. As the Father was living in Jesus, so is now the Spirit of God residing in the believers. This is the spiritual resemblance to our heavenly Father passed onto humankind since the beginning of creation.

> For in Christ all the fullness of the Deity lives in bodily
> form, and in Christ you have been brought to fullness.
> (Colossians 2:9,10)

Further, because we represent God, He charged us with the duty to participate with Him in the care of His creation. The Scripture tells us that,

> The LORD God took the man and put him in the Garden of
> Eden to work on it and care for it. (Genesis 2:15)

Two Hebrew words describe Adam's duties: lavodah (לעבדה) (root word: avad) "to work it" or "to care for it" and velshamrah (ולשמרה) (root word: shamar) "to guard it" or "to protect it." In the Old Testament, the Hebrew word avodah (עבדה) refers to the priestly duties of the Temple service. Similarly, Adam was tasked with serving God's creation in the same manner as the priests served in God's Temple. Before the Fall, the entire creation, unfettered from sin, represented God's Temple. The book of Revelation describes similar conditions in the new heaven and the new earth without a physical Temple "because the Lord God Almighty and the Lamb are its Temple." (Revelation 21:22).

Adam was also the guardian (shomer–שומר) of God's creation on earth, protecting the integrity of its holiness. One of God's names in the Scripture is Shomer Israel (שומר ישראל)—the Guardian of Israel–(Psalms 121:4) and comes from the same word root (shamar). God protects (שמר) those who love Him (Psalm 91:11; 121:5). As the Lord guards and protects His creation from heaven, so does Adam on earth. But what exactly was Adam guarding the Garden of Eden from? It was a perfect environment where Adam thrived, and God delighted in His creation. The Scripture informs us that the serpent, also known as Satan, had access to the Garden of Eden.

[Dragon's] tail swept a third of the stars out of the sky and flung them to the earth. ... The great dragon was hurled down —that ancient serpent called the devil, or Satan, who leads the whole world astray. He was hurled to the earth, and his angels with him (Revelation 12:4,9)

The serpent was already on earth, prior to Adam's creation. Adam's responsibility was to guard the Garden of Eden from the serpent. Adam failed. Humanity inherited this duty; we should also be seen as the guardians and protectors of God's creation from Satan. Just like Adam, we are failing in this divine commission. Nevertheless, this duty remains relevant today. The psalmist clearly declares, "The highest heavens belong to the Lord, but the earth he has given to man" (Psalms 115:16).

Humanity in The Created Order

The Scripture reveals God's intention for humanity when describing the position of mankind in God's created order.

> What is man that you are mindful of him, the son of man that you care for him. You have made him a little lower than the heavenly beings and crowned him with glory and honor. You made him ruler over the works of your hands; you put everything under his feet: all flocks and herds, and the beasts of the field, the birds of the air, and the fish of the sea, all that swim the paths of the seas. (Psalms 8:4-8)

The reference in verse 5, "You have made them a little lower than the heavenly beings," requires deeper study. The Hebrew root word used in "heavenly beings" is "Elohim" (אלהים), God Himself. Different Bible versions have translated "Elohim" (אלהים) differently: For example, "slightly less than divine" (CEB), "little lower than yourself" (CEV), "almost like gods" (ERV), "angels" (NIV, NCB, NCV, NKJV, KJV, TLV), or "God" (NASV, NLT, RSV, ASV, AMP). The prevailing translations view human beings as an intrinsic part of the divine order within the creation. God breathed the breath of life (His neshama, root word—נשמ) into Adam's nostrils, and he became a living being (Genesis 2:7). Since then, God's divine neshama has been passed on genealogically to each human being. When the divine origin of human beings is considered, the translation of this verse should say, "You have made them a little lower than God Himself." This elevates human beings to share in the same glory and honor that God possesses. His image and likeness, His glory and honor, have been passed on first to Adam and then to us. He is our Father. We bear His resemblance. He loves us. No wonder He died for us.

Similarly, the translation of verse 5b brings further clarification of the status given to humankind upon creation: "You crowned them with glory and honor." Glory (כבוד), translated in Hebrew, is "heaviness." It is an authority that weighs a lot, heavy with presence and respect. The Prophet Isaiah saw the glory (כבוד) "kevod" of God. In a dramatic vision, he describes seraphim, flying above God's throne, calling to one another in reverence:

> Holy, holy, holy is the LORD Almighty; the whole earth is full
>
> of his glory [כבוד]. (Isaiah 6:3)

God created Adam adorned with this same glory and honor. To rule and guard His creation, Adam had to have the same status and capability as God. This unique position in the created order gave Adam the authority to have dominion over God's creation.

The Roman Centurion displayed an astounding understanding of this order of authority in the spiritual realm. In the story (Matthew 8:5-13), Jesus called him a man of great faith and confirmed that this was the true spiritual order of things.

> When Jesus entered Capernaum, a centurion came to Him,
> asking for help. "Lord," he said, "my servant lies at home
> paralyzed, and in terrible suffering." Jesus said to him, "I will
> go and heal him." The centurion replied, "Lord, I do not
> deserve to have you come under my roof. But just say the

word, and my servant will be healed. For I myself am a man under authority with soldiers under me. I tell this one, 'Go,' and he goes; and that one, 'Come,' and he comes. I say to my servant, 'Do this,' and he does it." When Jesus heard it, He was astonished and said to those following him, "I tell you the truth, I have not found anyone in Israel with such great faith." (Matthew 8:5-13)

The Roman Centurion recognized the power and the authority Jesus had in the spiritual realm, metaphorically referring to the power and the authority he had over his subordinates in the natural realm.

Question: Do you recognize this spiritual authority? If so, does your prayer life reflect that understanding?

_____

_____

_____

_____

The Fall—The Loss of Authority

After the Fall, humankind lost its glory and honor, and with that, humankind lost the authority to govern matters on earth, as well. The authority didn't just vanish; it was stolen. Who took the authority after Adam failed? The Scripture tells us that through deceit, Satan comes to "steal, kill, and destroy" (John 10:10). The following text gives an understanding of this spiritual theft.

The devil led him up to a high place and showed him in an instant all the kingdoms of the world. And he said to him, "I will give you all their authority and splendor; it has been given to me, and I can give it to anyone I want to. If you worship me, it will all be yours." (Luke 4:5)

Jesus didn't argue with Satan about his statement of having all the authority on earth. He confronted him on the issue of worship, referring to Deuteronomy 6:13.

It is written: 'Worship the Lord your God and serve Him only.'
(Luke 4:8)

The authority was transferred to Satan, and humanity lost the glory (כבוד) "kevod" with which it was endowed upon creation. Jesus called Satan "the ruler of this world" (John 12:31; 14:30; 16:11).

Reinstatement of Authority and Power

On the cross, Jesus took back what Adam gave away and became the head over every power and authority (Colossians 2:10). The authority, divinely portioned to humankind at the beginning of creation, was reinstated. Jesus defeated the enemy and restored the rightful order of spiritual matters. At that moment in history, the authority was passed back from Satan to Jesus and through Jesus to all who believe in Him. Upon His ascension, Jesus passed His authority to His followers,

> Then Jesus came to them and said, "All authority in heaven and on earth has been given to me. Therefore, go and make disciples of all nations, baptizing them in the name of the Father and of the Son and of the Holy Spirit, and teaching them to obey everything I have commanded you. And surely I am with you always, to the very end of the age." (Matthew 28:18)

Jesus sent a group of seventy-two disciples into the community and gave them authority to minister to the people,

> I have given you authority to trample on snakes and scorpions and to overcome all the power of the enemy; nothing will harm you. (Luke 10: 17)

Jesus also gave His followers the authority to bind and release.

> Whatever you bind on earth will be bound in heaven, and whatever you loose on earth will be loosed in heaven. (Matthew 16:19)

This same authority is now ours. We are to "trample on snakes and scorpions" (Luke 10:19) without fear of harm. Scripture refers to demonic entities as snakes and scorpions. Jesus gave us the power and the authority to command them. He delivered on His promise on Pentecost.

> I will ask the Father, and he will give you another Counselor to
> be with you forever—the Spirit of truth. (John 14:16)

With this authority came the great commission: We are to make disciples of all nations (Matt 28:18). The restored authority comes with obligations. Adam's authority was to rule/guard God's creation; our authority is to resist Satan and expand God's Kingdom on earth by making disciples of all nations.

The authority and the power of prayer are granted in the inner room when we are one-on-one with God.

> But when you pray, go into your room, close the door, and
> pray to your Father, who is unseen. Then your Father, who
> sees what is done in secret, will reward you. (Matthew 6:6)

How do we pray, knowing we are endowed with such unique power and authority? Jesus redeemed, cleansed, sanctified, and vested His authority in us. We become His vessels on earth to do His will in heaven (Matthew 6:9-13). And yet, the real gain is not measured in authority units but in eternity units. Jesus responded to the overjoyed disciples:

> However, do not rejoice that the spirits submit to you, but
> rejoice that your names are written in heaven. (Luke 10:20)

According to Jesus, regaining authority is like gaining a lost territory on earth, but attaining His salvation is gaining eternal life forever and ever and ever in heaven. Believers must exercise God's power and authority to expand God's Kingdom on earth. Do you exercise this authority? We have been born in such a time as this to advance further God's plan for the complete redemption of humankind and nature until the new heaven and the new earth are established.

The Story of Adela

Adela was about to get married to a wonderful young man who was going through rigorous seminary training, preparing to be a pastor. Adela's commitment to her future husband compelled her to enroll in some seminary classes to prepare for their ministry. This is how, in that particular semester, Adela and her fiancé attended the same class with Dr. Garland, a professor and an ordained minister.

During class sessions, when Dr. Garland's eyes fell on Adela, he could hear the Lord's directives to bless her. There were other students with much more dire circumstances to attend to (at least from his perspective), so he responded to the Lord's nudging, "Yes, Lord, I will bless her." Before the semester ended, Dr. Garland finally had the opportunity to get together with Adela and pray for her. He faithfully laid hands over her, and being led by the Spirit, he decreed many blessings suitable for a woman of God. When he finished, Adela looked at him, her eyes full of tears. She assured him that these were tears of joy. Apparently, while Dr. Garland prayed over her, she saw two hands stretching over her head. These hands, she said, were not Dr. Garland's hands; these were Jesus' hands, she assured him. She was visually shaken as she described her vision during prayer. The hands were much larger, and the robe they were garbed in was white. At the time of the prayer, Dr. Garland was wearing a dark blue suit.

Dr. Garland was not less shaken and simultaneously deeply humbled because the Lord of heaven and earth, the Creator of the Universe, had chosen to use his hands as a conduit for His divine power and authority to bestow blessings on His people. Dr. Garland joined God to intervene in the state of affairs in His Creation. The dominion over God's creation given to Adam was now visibly demonstrated through the work of Dr. Garland. God partnered with him to accomplish His will on earth for Adela.

Sometimes, God lifts the veil of mystery, revealing His immediate participation in His creation. Adela's vision further solidified Dr. Garland's faith: The "nudge" was not his own imagination; it was God's directive to apply His authority, vested in Dr. Garland, to guard and rule His creation. What a wonderful partnership! Who said that the life of a believer is boring? Maturity in faith, becoming EHAD with God, increases the frequency of these experiences; they become a daily occurrence, building a recognizable pattern in the God-human relationship. We know His voice (John 10:27-28) and are elevated to the status of knowing God's business (John 15:15).

The story of Adela is a testimony to the power and authority in prayer. Our words are not a timid "breath" spoken in vain. They have the power to influence the spiritual realm. Our Lord, God, and Savior, Christ Jesus vested in us His power and authority. Jesus describes the mechanism through which His power and authority are employed through the believers to advance the Kingdom of God on earth.

> Don't you believe that I am in the Father and that the Father is in me? The words I say to you are not my own. Rather, it is the Father, living in me, who is doing his work. Believe me when I say that I am in the Father and the Father is in me; or at least believe on the evidence of the miracles themselves. I tell you the truth, anyone who has faith in me will do what I have been doing. He will do even greater things than these, because I am going to the Father. And I will do whatever you ask in my name, so that the Son may bring glory to the Father. You may ask me for anything in my name, and I will do it. (John 14:10-14)

A few things proceed from Jesus' words. **First**, the life of a follower of Christ should mirror the life of Jesus. He explained that anyone with faith in Him would do even "greater things." The only prerequisite for a believer to effect changes within the spiritual and physical realm, as Jesus did, is the presence of faith in Him. Our words of prayer spoken in faith can move mountains (Mark 11:23). Once spoken, they have a life of their own. They unfold, roll out, and progress through time, space, and realms until they deliver the desired results for which they were prayed. God's spoken word is effective.

> As the rain and the snow come down from heaven, and do not return to it without watering the earth and making it bud and flourish, so is my word that goes out from my mouth: It will not return to me empty, but will accomplish what I desire and achieve the purpose for which I sent it. (Isaiah 55:11)

Jesus said that our spoken words in faith in prayer should have the same effect. **Second**, signs and miracles accompanied Jesus' ministry, testifying of His power and authority over humanity and nature. Jesus said, "believe me on the account of the deeds." When spoken in faith, prayers produce deeds that speak for themselves. They are naturally supernatural. Physical laws are bent, and time and space are juxtaposed. The chasm between the natural and the spiritual realities is removed. The witnesses to these supernatural signs and miracles were bewildered, acknowledging that they had seen the acts of God.

> The people were all so amazed that they asked each other, "What is this? A new teaching—and with authority! He even gives orders to evil spirits, and they obey him." (Mark 1:27)

Nature and spirits obeyed Jesus because God the Father has given Him the authority (John 14:10). Consequently, nature and spirits should obey the believers because Jesus has endowed us with the same authority. The age of the apostles has never ended! God never withdrew His power and authority, but we have neglected our obligation to employ them in caring for and guarding His creation—humanity and nature.

Do you exercise power and authority in prayer to do God's will on earth, just like Dr. Garland did? This is faith in action. Believers should share daily personal testimonies of God's miracles in their lives. Encouraging one another increases faith. Miracles and faith mutually promulgate: Miracles increase faith; bigger faith results in more miracles. It is recorded in the Scripture that no miracles happened in Nazareth because of a lack of faith (Matthew 13:53–58). Pray that this is never our fate today.

Third, it is not through believers' exertion and effort that this unparalleled power and authority to command delivers astonishing results. The Father God bestowed His divine power and authority on Jesus. Jesus Himself testified, "It is the Father, living in me, who is doing his work" (John 14:10). The same divine power and authority Jesus gave to every believer (Luke 10:19). It is not the believer but Jesus living in the believer who performs the miracles. We are willing conduits for God to affect His creation. Faith is the only "must be present" catalyst to "officiate" a miraculous transaction. Blessed are those who have not seen and yet have believed (John 20:29). While Jesus was with the disciples, He gave them occasional power and authority. On Pentecost, upon His ascension, He sent the Holy Spirit to indwell believers with the same–but unlimited–power and authority.

Conclusion: Power is the state of indwelling with the Holy Spirit of every believer. It is given upon confession of faith in Jesus Christ as a personal Lord, God, and Savior. The Holy Spirit descends upon the individual, resurrecting the human spirit. Jesus referred to this as being born again (John 3:15). The spiritual Law decrees that every believer be sealed with the mark of the Holy Spirit (2 Corinthians 1:22; Ephesians 1:13; 4:30), assuring salvation. The indwelling of the Holy Spirit is the propeller of power in prayer. **Authority** is the right to employ this divine power of the Holy Spirit. Christ gave this right to those who believed in his name; He gave us the right to become children of God (John 1:12).

Restoration of the Creation to its Initial Glory

As we discussed earlier, Adam was endowed with power and authority upon his creation. The Fall resulted in the defilement of humankind and nature alike, upon which Adam lost all power and authority. Adam's transgression had an eternal consequence for the entire creation of God. Just like humankind, the creation was also defiled. It had to be redeemed and made perfect again. Jesus first came to redeem humankind through the cross. He will come again, this time to redeem nature and establish the new heaven and earth, the New Jerusalem. The Bible begins with a creation story and ends with a creation story.

> In the beginning, God created the heavens and the earth.
> (Genesis 1:1a)
> Then I saw a new heaven and a new earth, for the first heaven
> and the first earth had passed away. (Revelation 21:1)

The Prophet Isaiah foretold the second event.

> Behold, I will create new heavens and a new earth. The former
> things will not be remembered, nor will they come to mind.
> (Isaiah 65:17)

Why is there a need for a new heaven and a new earth? God created the first heaven and earth and deemed them as "very good" (Genesis 1:31). Nevertheless, we are told that God will create "new heaven and new earth" (Revelation 21:1–8). Why? The first creation suffered from the defilement of sin. Through Adam, sin entered not only humanity but also nature. While humanity suffered spiritual and physical death, nature entered an entropy mode. Entropy is the unfolding of the degradation of matter and energy within the universe that ultimately leads toward disorder and death. There were no floods, hurricanes, tornadoes, or earthquakes in Eden, and no illnesses or death. Adam and Eve were created immortals. They were allowed to partake of the Tree of Life and enjoyed immortality and the intimate presence of God. However, their access to the Tree of Life and to God was cut off upon the Fall (Genesis 3:24). Spiritual and physical death is, to this day, the fate of the human race. Jesus redeemed humanity from sin and death.

> Through Christ Jesus, the Law of the Spirit of life has set me
> free from the Law of sin and death. (Romans 8:2)

The redemption of nature is yet to come when the "new heaven and the new earth" will be established. Apostle Paul explains:

> The creation was subjected to frustration, not by its own choice, but because of the one who subjected it, in hope that the creation itself will be liberated from its bondage to decay and brought into the glorious freedom of the children of God. We know that the whole creation has been groaning as in the pains of childbirth right up to the present time.
> (Romans8:19-23)

The Fall affected the powers and authorities established at the beginning of time. The creation of the "new heaven and the new earth" restores these structures to their initial divine design.

The New Order of Things—The Message of Prophet Haggai

Since the Fall, God has been progressively revealing Himself to humanity. The magnitude of each revelation causes a fundamental shaking of the world's understanding of the spiritual order of things. The shaking is two-dimensional: Spiritual and physical. Each revelation is introduced on the foundation of a previous revelation. The New Testament cannot be understood without the Laws and the principles revealed in the Old Testament. The future of God's continuous revelations and interactions with humanity must be discerned and anticipated through the Old Writings.

> The secret things belong to the LORD our God, but the things revealed belong to us and to our children, that we may follow all the words of this Law. (Deuteronomy 29:29)

The death of Jesus on the cross in the New Testament cannot be understood without the sacrificial system elaborated in the Old Testament. The doctrines of forgiveness, redemption, peace, holiness, and salvation are not new doctrines; they are rather the old fundamentals, more clearly revealed at God's appointed time of the Messiah. God instructed us:

> Forget the former things; do not dwell on the past. See, I am
> doing a new thing! Now it springs up; do you not perceive it?
> (Isaiah 43:18-19a)

Each revelation shakes the core of humanity's understanding of the spiritual realm, and the world is never the same. The Word of the Lord through the Prophet Haggai records two of these fundamental shakings of "the heavens and the earth" (Haggai 2:6; 2:22). The author of the book of Hebrews builds on Haggai's prophecy and asserts that the phrase "I will once more shake the heavens and the earth" (Haggai 2:6) is predicated on a previous "shaking of heavens and the earth" which he asserts to have happened upon the giving of the Law on Mount Sinai (Hebrews 12:6).

The spiritual dimension of this first shaking of the heavens and the earth consists of the introduction of the monotheistic system of beliefs. Its stipulations, principles, and practices were in stark contrast to that era's polytheistic beliefs and practices; it rattled the spiritual worldviews and commonality of multiple god-worship within ancient nations. It established the sanctity of life and the holiness of living against the existing god-appeasing child sacrifices and detestable temple prostitution practices. It stipulated the laws of the halachic (kosher) lifestyle (from food to personal hygiene, from communal relationships to distinctive sacrificial and worship guidelines) as opposed to the existing defiling practices that are abominable in God's sight (Isaiah 66:3; Daniel 9:27;11:31; Revelation 17:5).

> Upon giving of the Law, the ground shook. On the morning of
> the third day there was thunder and lightening, with a thick
> cloud over the mountain, and very loud trumpet blast.
> Everyone in the camp trembled. Then Moses led the people
> out of the camp to meet with God, and they stood at the foot of
> the mountain. Mount Sinai was covered with smoke, because
> the LORD descended on it in fire. The smoke billowed up from

it like smoke from a furnace, and the whole mountain trembled violently. (Deuteronomy 19:17-19)

The writer of Hebrews attributed this event of physical manifestation to "his voice that shook the earth" (Hebrews 12:26a). Once the author of Hebrews established the fact of the first "shaking of the heavens and the earth," he then introduced the timeline of the second shaking.

"Once more I will shake not only the earth but also the heavens." The words "once more" indicate the removing of what can be shaken—that is, created things—so that what cannot be shaken may remain (Hebrews 12:26, 27).

In his discourse, the author of Hebrews refers to the incarnation of Jesus the Messiah, as the second shaking of the earth and heavens. The world is once again completely changed. He unfolds his argumentation on the prophecy of Haggai 2:6-9,

> This is what the LORD Almighty says: "In a little while, I will once more shake the heavens and the earth, the sea and the dry land. I will shake all nations, and the desired of all nations will come, and I will fill this house with glory," says the LORD Almighty. "The silver is mine, and the gold is mine," declares the LORD Almighty. "The glory of this present house will be greater than the glory of the former house," says the LORD Almighty. "And in this place, I will grant peace," declares the LORD Almighty. (Haggai 2:6-9)

The spiritual dimension of the second shaking introduced the New Covenant of Blood and Love to all humanity through the redemptive sacrifice of Jesus. It is a New Covenant of Blood because God's progressive revelation negated the existing sacrificial system, and instead, He offered Himself once and for all, "reconciling the world to Himself in Christ, not counting people's sins against them" (2 Corinthians 5:19). God Himself stepped into human history because

He saw that there was no one, he was appalled that there was no one to intervene; so his own arm achieved salvation for him, and his own righteousness sustained him. (Isaiah 59:16)

It is a New Covenant of Love because

God so loved the world that he gave his one and only Son, that whoever believes in him shall not perish but have eternal life. (John 3:16)

The victory on the Cross has universal spiritual "shaking"—it brought salvation to the Jews and the Gentiles alike. God Himself proclaims,

I will grant salvation to Zion, my splendor to Israel. (Isaiah 46:13b)

and also,

I will also make you a light for the Gentiles, that my salvation may reach to the ends of the earth. (Isaiah 49:6)

The victory on the Cross was also manifested by a physical shaking that occurred at the time of Jesus' death. Similarly to the physical shaking at Mount Sinai, the Bible recorded a shaking in the form of a powerful earthquake (Matthew 27:51) and darkness (Luke 23:44).

At that moment the curtain of the temple was torn in two from top to bottom. The earth shook, the rocks split, and the tombs broke open. The bodies of many holy people who had died were raised to life. They came out of the tombs after Jesus' resurrection and, went into the holy city and appeared to many people. (Matthew 27:51-53)

The author of Hebrews only discussed the "shaking of heaven and earth" in Haggai 2:6-9. However, there is another mention of the "shaking of heaven and earth" found in Haggai 2:21-23. Chapter 2 records two occasions when "the word of the Lord came through the Prophet Haggai" with the message of "shaking of heavens and earth." The first time was "on the twenty-first day of the seventh month" (Haggai 2:1). The second time was "on the twenty-fourth day of the ninth month, in the second year of Darius" (Haggai 2:10). The two messages of "shaking of heavens and the earth" are about two months apart but they appear to be prophecies of events that span two millennia apart. The first message is the prophecy of Jesus' incarnation when "the Word became flesh and made its dwelling among us" (John 1:1). The author of Hebrews discusses this event. This prophecy is now fulfilled. The second message appears to point at Jesus' second coming, a prophecy yet to be fulfilled.

The words in the second shaking of Haggai 2:21-22 are addressed to Zerubbabel and are infused with messianic meaning.

> "'Tell Zerubbabel governor of Judah that I am going to shake the heavens and the earth. I will overturn royal thrones, and I will shatter the power of the foreign kingdoms. I will overthrow chariots and their drivers; horses and their riders will fall, each by the sword of his brother.' " " 'On that day,' declares the LORD Almighty, 'I will take you, my servant Zerubbabel son of Shealtiel,' declares the LORD, 'and I will make you like my signet ring, for I have chosen you,' declares the LORD Almighty." (Haggai 2:21-23)

Examination of the second "shaking of the heaven and earth" message indicates a complete overthrow of the existing world's political system (royal thrones and foreign kingdoms) and military system (chariots and their drivers, horses and their riders). There will be such strife within families that brothers will slay each other by their own swords (v.22b). The words "overturn" or "overthrow" (הפךְ), "destroy" (שמד) and again "overturn" or "overthrow" (הפךְ) are a configuration of triple warning, a literary feature in Scripture, referring to assurance of events to come—utter destruction and annihilation. The same Hebrew word "overturn or overthrow" (הפךְ) describes the destruction of Sodom and Gomorrah. The devastation recorded in both texts illustrates a total annihilation of an existing place, as described in Genesis 18:16-19:29 and

Haggai 2:22,23. Jesus Himself spoke of such a time of destruction as a sign of His second coming.

> Nation will rise against nation, and kingdom against kingdom.
> There will be famines and earthquakes in various places.
> (Matthew 24:7)

Jesus equated these political and military turmoils with birth pains (Matthew 24:8). The physical shaking will be so intense that Jesus warned us of those days in advance.

> For then, there will be great distress, unequaled from the beginning of the world until now—and never to be equaled again. (Matthew 24:21)

The words of Jesus and the writing of the Prophet Haggai appear to be referring to a third "shaking of heaven and earth" that will happen upon the second coming of Jesus. The physical shaking is the cosmic cataclysm that will occur upon the creation of the new heavens and the new earth. Jesus spoke of earthly and heavenly cataclysmic events, declaring,

> Immediately after the distress of those days, the sun will be darkened, and the moon will not give its light; the stars will fall from the sky, and the heavenly bodies will be shaken. (Matthew 24:29)

When speaking about these cataclysms, Jesus pointed to the Day of the Lord prophesied by Isaiah, Ezekiel, Joel, Amos, Obadiah, Zephaniah, Zechariah, and Malachi. The spiritual significance of those days is referred to as Judgement Day, when everyone will be judged for what they have done (Romans 2:6). Those who rejected Jesus will go away to eternal punishment, but the righteous to eternal life (Matthew 25:46).

Haggai spoke to Zerubbabel (2:2, 21), the governor of Judah at that historic time. The main message of his prophecy urged the people who returned from the Babylonian exile to no longer delay the rebuilding of the temple of God in Jerusalem. This is the second temple that will last 420 years. It is a temple in which only Jews had access to the inner courts of worship. Gentiles were relegated to the outer court. Yet, through Haggai, God spoke of a temple for all nations. God declared that in His temple, "the desired of all nations will come, and I will fill this house with glory," says the LORD Almighty (Haggai 2:7).

Even more, God declared that "the glory of this present house (the redeemed in Jesus) will be greater than the glory of the former house (physical temple)," and "in this place, I will grant peace" (in the heart of the believers in Jesus) (Haggai 2:9). It is the community of believers in Jesus that constitutes God's temple where His glory dwells now. Apostle Paul writes in his letter to the Corinthians,

> Don't you know that you yourselves are God's temple and that
> God's Spirit lives in you? If anyone destroys God's temple,
> God will destroy him; for God's temple is sacred, and you are
> that temple. (1 Corinthians 3:16-17)

Haggai's message speaks of the current and former glory of God's temple (Haggai 2:9); Isaiah's message speaks of new and former things (Isaiah 43:18-19). This weaving through now and then, between the current and the prophetic, is an example of what Jesus often referred to, "Let the reader understand" (Matthew 24:15), or "Whoever has ears let them hear" (Matthew 13:9;13:43;23:35; Luke 8:8;14:35; Mark 4:9). He very often spoke about the spiritual order of things openly and truthfully. Our minds, however, tend to superimpose our three-dimensional, time-based physical reality on His out-of-this-world spiritual truths. When Jesus said, "Very truly I tell you, unless you eat the flesh of the Son of Man and drink his blood, you have no life in you" (John 6:53), He angered His audience because the halachic (kosher) laws forbid Jews to consume blood and—God forbid—human flesh. Jesus, however, referred to the meaning of His sacrifice on the Cross for forgiveness of sins and the meaning of the Eucharist. When Jesus spoke of "destroy this temple, and I will raise it again in three days" (John 2:19), He referred to His crucifixion and resurrection on the third day. Jesus spoke to the people with parables because,

> The knowledge of the secrets of the kingdom of heaven has been given to you [with ears to hear and eyes to see and understand the spiritual realm], but not to them [those who do not yet have spiritual discernment]. (Matthew 13:11)

Similarly, Haggai's text speaks simultaneously to the people during the former temple period and to the believers in Jesus as the temple of the living God now. Haggai simultaneously spoke to the governor of Judea, Zerubbabel, and to us, whose bodies are now the living temple of God. These examples are known in English as a literary device of metaphorical symbolism—using double levels of meaning for the exact words or expressions. In the Bible, the meanings are determined by the chronological order of the biblical events they depict. The last verse of Haggai's message is a crescendo—a powerful display of this literary feature, depicting a prophecy for the times yet to come. Haggai is instructed to tell Zerubbabel that,

> 'On that day,' declares the LORD Almighty, 'I will take you, my servant Zerubbabel son of Shealtiel,' declares the LORD, 'and I will make you like my signet ring, for I have chosen you,' declares the LORD Almighty. (Haggai 2:23)

The expression "on that day" in the Scripture always refers to future messianic events. Second, the Lord refers to Zerubbabel as His servant. In the Bible, the office of a servant always refers to a messianic figure. Zerubbabel was commissioned to build the second temple; Jesus' mission was to build the eternal temple of God, indwelling within His holy people. The new order of things through Jesus the Messiah negated the old sacrificial practices of the physical temple and made it obsolete. Instead, the redeemed in Jesus become the embodiment of the eternal temple of God. The first temple built by hands has now passed away, overridden by the eternal temple of God's holy people. In the context of the previous verse (Haggai 2:22), the cataclysmic events are followed by the return of Jesus the Messiah when,

> All the nations of the earth will mourn. They see the Son of Man coming on the clouds of the sky with power and great glory. And then he will send his angels with a loud trumpet call, and they will gather his elect from the four winds, from one end of the heavens to the other. (Matthew 24:30)

The meaning of the name Zerubbabel (זרבבל) means "the one sown in Babylon," "begotten in Babylon," or "conceived in captivity." The seed of Zerubbabel had the yeast of Babylon, a scriptural symbol of captivity and evil. It was subjected to decay and destruction. Through Jesus, however, that same seed, begotten under the captivity of Babylon, is now being redeemed and made indestructible for all eternity, forever and ever. The final words to Zerubbabel are also words to the redeemed in Jesus,

> "'I will take you, my servant, Zerubbabel son of Shealtiel,' declares the LORD." (Haggai 2:23)

They are reiterations of Jesus' own words with which He comforted His disciples upon the news of His departure,

> And if I go and prepare a place for you, I will come back and take you to be with me that you also may be where I am. (John 14:3)

The signet ring is a royal symbol. It is the stamp of the authority of the King. God gives His authority and mark of approval to Zerubbabel. In the messianic context of the text, God also gives His authority to all His redeemed because,

> He anointed us, set His seal of ownership on us, and put His Spirit in our hearts as a deposit, guaranteeing what is to come. (2 Corinthians 1:22)

And the Lord our God will do this because we are a chosen people, a royal priesthood, a holy nation, God's special possession (1 Peter 2:9).

How great is the love the Father has lavished on us that we should be called children of God! (1 John 3:1)

The messianic significance of Haggai 2:22,23 has an urgent implication for us today. It comes through the third reference of the "shaking of heaven and earth." Jesus warned us to be on guard and gave us specific signs to recognize the times when these prophesied events would occur. The prophecy of His second coming is yet to be fulfilled.

Testimony of Pastor Tom

Recently, upon studying the books of Hebrews and Haggai, the expression "shaking of the heaven and the earth" drew my attention. I pursued the Lord's lead and came to a deeper understanding of the three "shakings of heaven and earth." The Lord "opened" my mind to "see" the spiritual meaning of Haggai 2:6 and 2:21 as the Prophetic unfolding of His first and second coming. He simultaneously brought to my mind, along with His own words, "the heavenly bodies will be shaken" (Matthew 24:29), a personal experience with Him. Jesus' prophetic words were superimposed on a dream He gave me ten years earlier. The dream is consistent with the message of the Scripture; it doesn't add or take away from the scriptural text but magnifies its meaning, making it significant for today's times. Here is my eyewitness account of the supernatural experience of being taught by the finger of God.

That night, I had a dream. In my dream, I woke up and sat in my bed, my wife soundly asleep beside me. I looked toward our second-story balcony and saw a strange sight: The sun was going with incredible speed into sunrise– sunset mode; it was moving from rising to setting positions in seconds. For a long moment, I sat in bed, mesmerized by the incredibly fast-paced cycle of the sun. Then, I woke up, and I knew it was a dream from the Lord. At the time of this experience, the level of my spiritual maturity enabled me to distinguish between the dreams of the flesh and the dreams from God. This was a dream from God. I immediately asked the Lord about the meaning of the dream, and brushing it away as "too bizarre," I soon went back to sleep. That morning, during my quiet time with the Lord, I inquired of the meaning of the dream. "I don't understand, Lord," I groaned as I tried to make sense of the experience.

The very next night, the dream repeated. Again, in my dream, I woke up, sitting on the bed, watching the sun rise and set with the same incredible speed, but this time, I was taken into outer space. From far beyond our solar system, I saw celestial bodies moving chaotically. Compared to them, the earth was very, very tiny, and it was spinning out of control. Many stellar structures came dangerously close to causing a collision. One particularly massive formation with no spherical shape was on a collision trajectory with the earth. The impact scraped the surface of earth, and I heard a terrifying cosmic sound that resembled the scraping of metal-on-metal surfaces but on a much larger, cosmic scale. I put my hands to my ears to lessen the pain from the sound, and I cried out, "Lord, there are people down there who are hurt." Immediately, I was taken down to earth into an apartment building. A woman, alone in her flat, was packing a suitcase, piling items randomly. She was not in a hurry, neither scared nor distressed. The building began to sway—an earthquake was occurring, but again, I saw no urgency in the woman's demeanor. She got down on street level. No shops were open. Everything appeared deserted. Bands of vehicles, full of troubled people, swooshed by, hurrying north (an impression I got). The woman's intentions were the same as she picked up the panic. Suddenly, I was taken up in the cosmic realm again, looking intensely at the heavenly bodies as they were shaken. And then, back to earth. The same picture —everything in our universe was spinning out of control, and there was panic on earth. Then I woke up.

I immediately understood—the Lord answered my inquiry from the day before. Jesus' words, "the heavenly bodies will be shaken" (Matthew 24:29b), were engraved in my mind. I understood that the seconds-long sunrises and sunsets were caused by the out-of-control spinning of the earth, which the Lord clearly showed me. The physical Law of gravity no longer held sway in this apocalyptic dream. I went to Scripture for further guidance. And I understood: Jesus was referring to His second coming.

> The sun will be darkened, and the moon will not give its light; the stars will fall from the sky, and the heavenly bodies will be shaken. (Matthew 24:29-31)

Jesus showed me these cataclysmic events. They are the signs of His second coming; the sign of the Son of Man appearing in heaven (Matthew 24:31). The Prophet Isaiah reiterated the same apocalyptic message.

> The LORD Almighty has a day in store for all the proud and lofty, for all that is exalted. The arrogance of man will be brought low and human pride humbled. People will flee to caves in the rocks and to holes in the ground from the fearful presence of the LORD and the splendor of his majesty, when he rises to shake the earth. (Isaiah 2:12-22)

Throughout the years, I continued reflecting on this dream, and an understanding formed—it depicted the world after the rapture, just as Jesus had described it to His disciples (Matthew 24:29). There were very few people. I didn't see any children. It appeared that natural disasters like earthquakes have become a "daily" experience, judging by the woman's demeanor—for her, the shaking of the building seemed "normal." The most horrifying sight was the celestial chaos and the fact that there were still people on earth who had been left behind. I saw their demise, and my heart grew heavy.

When the consistency of the Scripture spans over the writings of the Old and the New Testaments, it grabs the believer's attention with an augmented message. When a personal experience of dream or vision is consistent with the message of the Scripture, the voice of the Lord God becomes louder and clearer. His message rises above the noise of life and stands strong against any doubts:

"Tell everyone I am coming and will not delay" (Hebrews 10:37). I didn't shout His message from the rooftops but have been telling everyone on my path—first to my family, then to friends, and even strangers. Recipients of His message are the community of believers because His Word is God-breathed and is useful for "teaching, rebuking, correction, and training in righteousness" (2 Timothy 3:16). I cannot but speak of His revelation with boldness because

> His Word is in my heart like a fire, a fire shut up in my bones.
>
> I am weary of holding it down; indeed, I cannot. (Jeremiah 20:9)

This message is more urgent today than it was ten years ago. We are closer to the fulfillment of Haggai 2:22-23—Jesus' second coming. At the rapture, He is taking to Himself all those conceived in Babylon but redeemed through His blood. He is coming back a second time to judge the world. You don't want to be on earth then, finding yourself on the wrong side of eternity.

As of the time I wrote about my dream, rapture has not happened yet. Let us all pray that our lamps are full with oil as we diligently wait for our bridegroom (Matthew 25:1-13). He is coming and will not delay. Keep watch because you don't know the day or the hour.

EHAD with GOD

REFLECTION—Week Two

Reflection 1: Give Him Five (5 minutes)—the daily practice of God's presence (see description on pages 41 and 63 under "Deep calls to deep" section)

Reflection 2: Daily confession and repentance in prayer to Christ—our high priest; crucify the flesh, wash with the blood, fill with the Holy Spirit (page 13)

Reflection 3: The Story of Rose: Manifestation of the practices of the flesh

The Story of Rose

Rose was ecstatic. Her prayers for the job she had long desired were finally granted. She immediately got on the task of acquiring a new wardrobe. Ross, known as the "dress for less" store, appealed to her taste and budget. Entering the store, she didn't take a cart. Instead, as she moved through the rows, she began piling clothing over her shoulder, still with the hangers. As a woman passed in the opposite direction, one of the hangers caught a piece of the woman's merchandise. Rose playfully stepped backward to release the hanger, quietly chuckling at the funny situation. She turned to face and apologized to the woman, and for a quick moment, both women locked eyes. Rose's apologetic smile froze at the sight of the woman's eyes gushing hatred and disgust at her. "How dare you do such an awful thing!" the woman's ice-cold demeanor shouted at her. In that blink of an eye, Rose saw deep in the woman's soul and her heart ached. Her smiling eyes now flowed with empathy towards this stranger. Beneath the nice appearance, Rose saw a deeply wounded individual. The woman lowered her eyes, realizing the absurdity of her reaction to such an insignificant situation: The punishment (level of hatred) was greater than the "hanger" crime.

Both women parted ways. One with prayer on her lips for the soul in pain she just encountered; the other with disgust with herself for allowing a stranger to see what she has been guarding for a long time. The woman thought she had locked her heart to the pain and had thrown the key away, but the ugly head of pain had found its way to the surface in the mutant form of anger and hate. And it was supposed to be just a mundane task of shopping.

Task: Recall a situation when you have responded with an inadequate reaction. What triggered your reaction? Did the conflict find you unprepared? How often is your response to mundane situations "out of proportion?"

_____
_____
_____
_____
_____
_____
_____
_____
_____
_____

The woman's reaction is a manifestation of a deep underlying problem that had taken root in her heart and mind. Anger and hatred are just the visual manifestations of the woman's root problem: Her spirit was marred. Jesus explained:

> A good man [woman] brings good things out of the good
> stored up in his [her] heart, and an evil man [woman] brings
> evil things out of the evil stored up in his [her] heart. For out
> of the overflow of the heart, the mouth speaks. (Luke 6:45)

Anger and hatred don't belong to the Kingdom of God. These are the evil things stored up in her heart that Jesus referred to; these are the practices of the flesh that manifest in anger and hate. Let's examine ourselves and identify areas in our lives where we have sown a bad seed and have reaped a bad fruit (Galatians 6:7).

Task: List practices of the flesh that have a stronghold over your life. How do these practices affect your life?

_____
_____
_____
_____
_____
_____
_____
_____
_____
_____
_____
_____

Do you desire to liberate yourself from the oppressive presence of these practices? Keep moving on the narrow road for EHAD with GOD, and you will be set free.

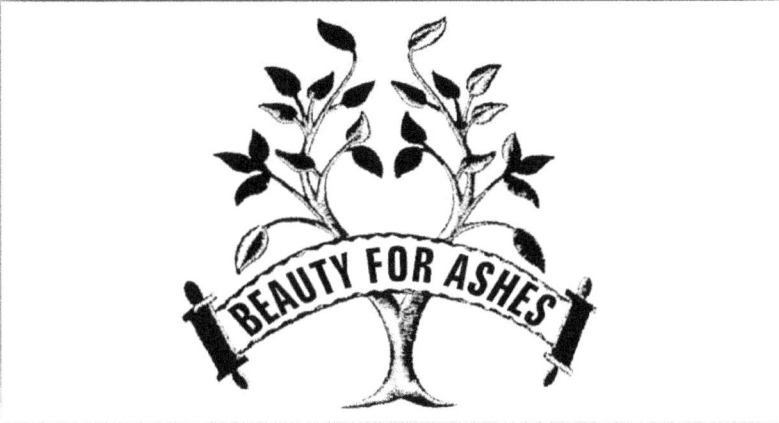

SESSION THREE

THE LAW OF GOD

Why do we turn attention to the Law of God for healing from traumatic events and spiritual oppression? It is very simple: The process of healing the human soul is the process of making one right with God. How do I know I am in right standing with God? It is when I satisfy God's requirements for righteous living, becoming EHAD with God. The Law of God is the divine manual for righteous living under the fallen conditions of this world. It postulates spiritual guidelines for attitudes and behaviors with God and people that are universal. The elaborate 613 Old Testament laws and precepts directed people from that era to live righteously with God. Yet, the Scripture declares that,

> There is no one righteous, not even one; there is no one who
> understands; there is no one who seeks God. All have turned
> away, they have together become worthless; there is no one
> who does good, not even one. (Romans 3:10-12)

This is the curse of the Law of God. No human can meet the righteous requirements of the Law. Jesus, God Himself, came to redeem humanity from

97

this curse. Only through faith in Him is the believer granted the capacity to meet the righteous requirements of the Law of God. The impartation of the Holy Spirit sanctifies the whole spirit, soul, and body, making the believer blameless (1 Thessalonians 5:23). The prophets Jeremiah and Ezekiel foretold of this marvelous transformation.

> "This is the covenant I will make with the people of Israel
> after that time," declares the Lord. "I will put my law in
> their minds and write it on their hearts. I will be their God,
> and they will be my people. (Jeremiah 31:33)
> I will give them an undivided heart and put a new spirit in
> them; I will remove from them their heart of stone and
> give them a heart of flesh. (Ezekiel 11:19)
> I will give you a new heart and put a new spirit in you; I
> will remove from you your heart of stone and give you a
> heart of flesh. (Ezekiel 36:26)

God didn't lower His standards for righteous living. He enabled humanity to live up to the righteous requirements of the Law by imparting His own righteousness, holiness, and goodness through a simple faith in Jesus.

The Law of God—The Foundation of Life in Fullness

Human beings, being made after God's image, integrate in themselves the physical (body) and the spiritual (soul and spirit) realms of God's creation.

> The LORD God formed the man from the dust of the ground
> [physical realm] and breathed into his nostrils the breath of
> life [spiritual realm], and the man became a living being.
> (Genesis 2:7)

Even before God created the first man, God created the physical means for his survival. The provision for life's necessities assured the support of physical life through that same realm.

Then God said, "I give you every seed-bearing plant on the face of the whole earth and every tree that has fruit with seed in it. I give every green plant for food." And it was so. (Genesis 1:29-30)

However, life in wholeness and health is not solely sustained by the provision for Adam's physical needs. Such oversight would have neglected an intrinsic part of his nature, his soul and spirit. God's assurance for life in wholeness also included provision for his spiritual needs. God Himself was the source of spiritual sustenance. Adam was allowed into the presence of God, and there was nothing to hinder their relationship. He walked in the garden in the cool of the day, remaining under God's blessing, seeing and hearing God, and enjoying His fellowship (Genesis 3:8-10). With the Fall, though, Adam lost all. He was cut off from the very source of life that sustained his spiritual and physical health. The entire human race inherited this condition. Return to the original divine design is only possible through faith in Christ.

The sovereignty of God as Creator is visible through the things and the beings He created. His stamp of divine craftsmanship is displayed by supreme intelligence behind the diversity of life forms and the unmatchable conditions for their existence within the vast dimensions of time and space. There is a perfection of unity, integration, and interdependence between the creation's smallest and greatest elements and between the living and the nonliving. The core of this balance is based on God's irreversible physical (natural) and spiritual laws.

With the creation of the first man, the physical and the spiritual realms became integrated, coming into existence on full display. God is Spirit; angels and demons are spirits also. Only humankind integrates the physical and spiritual realities in a living form. Demon oppression and possession are a hijacking of the human faculties so that demons experience the pleasure of life through the human senses, which they otherwise don't have. Since they are evil creatures, the oppressed people exhibit evil behavior, causing them to trespass

God's Law, assigning them a condemnation to hell. During His earthly ministry, Jesus broke the chains of many oppressed people, such as Mary Magdalene (Luke 8:2) and the demon-possessed man in Gerasenes (Mark 5:1-20; Luke 8:26-39). Jesus was accused of associating with sinners, but He responded:

> It is not the healthy who need a doctor, but the sick. I have not
> come to call the righteous, but sinners. (Mark 2:17)

Jesus had compassion and empathy, not condemnation for those oppressed by evil forces. The story of the woman at the well (John 4:1-42) and the story of the woman caught in adultery (John 8:3:11) are biblical narratives that exemplify His heart for the downtrodden. Our attitude toward them should also model empathy and compassion, not hatred and condemnation. Yet, we should never depart from the spiritual truth that freedom from oppression is only possible when the evil spirits, who exhibit the vile behavior through the oppressed person, must be evicted and expelled. Spiritual deliverance must include the full cooperation of the victim. Knowledge of spiritual reality is a must so that people can make informed decisions about their eternal destiny in heaven or hell and agree with the process of deliverance. The Church must preach and teach the truth in love; it is a divinely assigned responsibility to care for God's creation. This is the way of love which Jesus taught. *EHAD with GOD* teaches the same way to freedom through self-deliverance.

The preservation of human life was assured under one condition: Human beings would acknowledge and obey the natural and spiritual laws that governed the realms. Natural laws govern the material world within which humans live. Life on earth runs according to the precise and irrevocable functioning of these laws that continue to sustain the existence of life to this day. Spiritual laws govern the spiritual realm. They are God's standard for moral living and prescribe the ways for sustained spiritual health. Since the beginning, the physical realm has been governed by numerous natural laws, like the law of gravity and the laws of thermodynamics, for example. They are mere descriptions of the way the world functions. God, however, gave only one law to govern the spiritual realm. The Lord God commanded man not to eat from the Tree of Knowledge of Good and Evil (Genesis 2:17).

After the Fall, the number of physical laws remained the same while the number of spiritual laws drastically increased: From one, they became ten—the Ten Commandments (Deuteronomy 5:6-21). This tenfold increase[3] was necessary to preserve humans' spiritual life under the fallen conditions. The trespassing of the spiritual law resulted in a drastic deterioration of humans' standing with God: From being a "very good" creation (Genesis 1:31), humanity turned into an object destined to destruction (Genesis 6:7). The rapid deterioration was caused by alienation from God. Adam, Eve, and their offspring could no longer live according to the righteous requirements of the spiritual laws. They became corrupted.

God expelled Adam and Eve from The Garden of Eden (Genesis 3:23), which consequently placed their life in a dangerous situation. Without God's presence, they were now exposed relentlessly to devious deceptions and crafty manipulations of Satan. Their disobedience gave the Devil a foothold (Ephesians 4:27) to lodge himself into the human soul and manipulate the mind. Under these conditions, the seed of sin grew rapidly and manifested itself through the escalation of humans' wickedness: Cain's anger (Genesis 4:5) speedily led to the premeditated act of Abel's brutal murder (Genesis 4:5,8).

The Ten Commandments are the power God gave humans to counteract the evil influence of the Devil. The Mosaic Law is a God-given guide to practice God's presence under the fallen condition. Obedience to these laws assured that the human spirit would remain alive; humans would retain their human nature and restore their position for close fellowship with God, ultimately becoming once again EHAD with God, receiving "fullness in Christ" (Colossians 2:10). Sin

---

3 Between these two events are also the Noahide Laws given to all humanity after the Flood.

is a transgression against God's Law (1 John 3:4). Holiness, then, is conformity to God's Law (Romans 7:12).

God never needed to clarify any of His physical laws, but throughout human history, He continuously revealed His spiritual commandments through the Bible. Their significance is the subject matter throughout the Old and New Testaments. The Bible teaches to choose life through obedience to God's Law (Deuteronomy 30:19). It offers free redemption through Jesus, the Messiah (John 3:10). It conveys the core truth about the healing of the human soul, body, and spirit (1 Thessalonians 5:23).

The Israelites recognized the importance of God's Law by making it a central part of their governing system. The early rabbinic tradition, known as the Oral Torah, acknowledges the supremacy of the spiritual laws over the physical laws and teaches that God looked into the Torah (the Law) and created the world. He designed the universe to make it possible for human beings to carry out the commandments[4]. God created humans with the full capacity to measure up to God's holy standard.

Today, we continue to reap the consequences of Adam's disobedience. Even more, despite the advantage of the abundant historical and biblical narrative from which to learn, we continue to ignore God's warning that disobedience to His spiritual laws is sin and the wages of sin is death (Romans 6:23a).

The Way of Life and the Way of Death

God, who is Spirit, cannot be seen and experienced through physical sight and touch. Because the laws of God are spiritual, they must be obeyed in faith; what God has spoken is to be accepted as His ultimate Word of divine truth to us.

---

[4] Rabbi Nosson Scherman, The Chumash, The Torah: Haftaros and Five Megillos With a Commentary Anthologized from the Rabbinic Writings, The Stone Edition, The ArtScroll Series (Brooklyn, NY: Mesorah Publications, 2000), xxi.

In the story of the rich man and Lazarus (Luke 16:19-31), the rich man's defiance assigned him a place in Hell. He begged Abraham to send Lazarus back to his five brothers, so they would repent and not come to the place of torment where he found himself. Abraham replied,

> They have Moses and the Prophets; let them listen to them.
>
> (Luke 16:29)

The Apostle Peter also implored us to recall the words spoken in the past by the holy prophets and the command given by our Lord and Savior through the Apostles (2 Peter 3:2). We are instructed to trust the Word of God and accept its authority. The Lord God declared through His servant, the Prophet Habakkuk that "the righteous will live by his faith" (Habakkuk 2:4b). And Jesus Himself reiterated the importance of faith,

> Blessed are those who have not seen and yet have believed.
>
> (John 20:29)

Preserving humans' physical existence is grounded in the acknowledgment and obedience to all physical laws. The Lord equipped us with the senses and intelligence to recognize, accept, live, obey, and survive according to these laws. We have learned never to question the law of gravity, the consequences of prolonged exposures to high or low temperatures, or the consumption of toxic chemical substances. Preserving life requires unquestionable respect for these laws as an assurance for survival. Violation of even a fraction of these laws results in physical harm or even death.

In complete contrast to the unquestionable obedience to the natural laws is humans' long history of disobedience to the spiritual laws. Adam and Eve disobeyed God's commandment and sin and death entered humanity.

> Sin entered the world through one man, and death through
>
> sin, and in this way death came to all men, because all sinned.
>
> (Romans 5:12)

The Bible records a similar destiny for Ephraim; the moment he offended through Baal worship, he died (Hosea 13:1). Death in the above cases refers to spiritual death. Baal worship broke the first commandment: You shall have no other gods before me (Deuteronomy 5:7). The blessings and curses, life and death for obeying or disobeying God's Laws refrain throughout the Bible. The Prophet declared,

> Say to them, 'As surely as I live, declares the Sovereign LORD, I take no pleasure in the death of the wicked, but rather that they turn from their ways and live. Turn! Turn from your evil ways! Why will you die, O house of Israel?' (Ezekiel 33:11)

The Prophet Ezekiel speaks to the Israelites of spiritual death due to sin. Only turning away from their corrupt ways can cancel their spiritual death. The Prophet Isaiah reminds them about the consequences of disobeying the Law: The land suffers from being defiled by the abominable practices of humans.

> The earth is defiled by its people; they have disobeyed the laws, violated the statutes, and broken the everlasting covenant. Therefore, a curse consumes the earth; its people must bear their guilt. (Isaiah 24:5,6)

In the book of Revelation, Jesus sternly warns the church in Sardis. He identified their problem as spiritual death.

> I know your deeds; you have a reputation of being alive, but you are dead. (Revelation 3:1)

Apostle Paul sternly warns,

> For if you live according to the flesh, you will die; but if by the Spirit you put to death the misdeeds of the body, you will live. (Romans 8:13)

The death that results from disobedience to God's spiritual laws is spiritual. Are the believers shielded from such finality? Do we view our position in the Kingdom of God as so privileged that we can override God's spoken Word and His spiritual Law? Are we victims of the enemy's deceit, or is it just our foolishness? A willful disregard for Jesus' words may lead to the predicament faced by the church of Sardis. We, the believers, must "wake up and strengthen what remains and is about to die" (Revelation 3:1).

The Blessing and The Curse

The giving of the Law came with a blessing and a curse. Because the Law is spiritual, so are the consequences of obeying or disobeying it. Obedience to the Law evokes great blessings; disobedience is a curse.

> The earth is defiled by its people; they have disobeyed the laws, violated the statutes, and broken the everlasting covenant. Therefore, a curse consumes the earth; its people must bear their guilt. (Isaiah 24:5-6)

When we operate under blessings, we are in compliance with the laws governing the natural and spiritual realms; we obey these laws and thrive. But when we engage in sin, we place ourselves under a curse. Then, the irrevocable Word of God is executed, making all the curses of the Bible come true in our lives.

The giving of the Law placed Israel in a covenantal relationship with God. It came with a life and death offer. The Lord took extraordinary steps to introduce it to the Israelites. Moses proclaimed and sealed with words in the ears of the Israelites the significance of accepting God's Law:

> You have declared this day that the LORD is your God and that you will walk in His ways, that you will keep his decrees, commands, and laws, and that you will obey him. And the LORD has declared this day that you are his people, his treasured possession as he promised, and that you are to keep all His commands. (Deuteronomy 26:17-18)

To further emphasize the absolute importance of His spiritual laws with their life-and-death consequences, the Lord God gave thorough instructions to the Israelites through Moses:

> When you cross the Jordan, half of the tribes shall stand
> on Mount Gerizim to bless the people, and half of the
> tribes shall stand on Mount Ebal to pronounce the curses
> of the Law (Deuteronomy 27:12-13).

The blessings and the curses were part of the agreement made under God's covenant (Deuteronomy 28:1-13). The instructions were clear: If you fully obey the Lord your God and carefully follow all his commands, you will be blessed. You will always be at the top, never at the bottom (Deuteronomy 28:1-14). The passage is a long list of the physical and spiritual blessings that will surely come with obedience to God's Law. In contrast, the Scripture describing the curses is terrifying.

> However, if you do not obey the LORD your God and do not
> carefully follow all his commands and decrees, all these curses
> will come upon you and overtake you (Deuteronomy 28:15).

The list of physical and spiritual curses that follow is much more exhaustive than the one describing the blessings. Even more, the warnings of the curses due to disobedience of the Law are written twice (Deuteronomy 27:15-26; 28:15-68)!

Life and Death Offer

To assure clarity of the covenantal relationship, Moses summoned the Israelites twice, once in Horeb and again in Moab, teaching them the terms of the covenant. The Lord God Himself appealed to the Israelites:

> See, I set before you today life and prosperity, death
> and destruction. ... This day, I call heaven and earth as
> witnesses against you that I have set before you life and
> death, blessings and curses. Now choose life, so that
> you and your children may live. (Deuteronomy
> 30:15-19)

The blessings and the curses are embedded in the Law. It is a life or death offer, and there is no middle ground. Acceptance or disobedience sets into motion forces that the Word of the Almighty God preordained and thus is irrevocable. Redemption and restoration from disobedience are also feasible provisions of the same Law.

> When you and your children return to the LORD your God and obey him with all your heart and with all your soul ... then the LORD your God will restore your fortunes and have compassion on you. (Deuteronomy 30:2-3)

Our God is a Holy God! When the continuous practice of sin defiles a person, when there is no repentance, God withdraws His presence and has nothing to do with the calamities that follow. The realm without God is under the authority of Satan (Luke 4:6). This is what God says to such people:

> Then I will go back to my place until they admit their guilt. And they will seek my face; in their misery, they will earnestly seek me. (Hosea 5:15)

Just like the Israelites entered into a covenantal relationship with God on Mount Sinai, so is every person who makes a profession of faith in Christ. The believers commit to obedience to God's Law and assume all responsibilities for not keeping their end of the covenant. Jesus explained to the disciples,

> Anyone who loves me will obey my teaching. My Father will love them, and we will come to them and make our home with them. Anyone who does not love me will not obey my teaching. (John 14:23,24)

How many times have we sighed in distress, blaming God for the evil He supposedly had allowed in our lives? According to the Scripture, it is not God but our own doing that evokes the curses of the Law. Are we, as Christians, who Christ redeemed from the curse of the Law by becoming a curse for us (Galatians 3:13), exempt from triggering the curses when we sin? The Apostle Paul is clear, "Absolutely not!" (Romans 6:1, 15). The Law doesn't oppose the promises of God (Galatians 3:21). Jesus consistently taught in the same manner.

> Do not think that I have come to abolish the Law or the
> Prophets; I have not come to abolish them but to fulfill them.
> (Matthew 5:17)

The curses and the blessings are part of God's covenant. They were, are, and will continue to be in power, accomplishing their purposes as surely as God lives. We, like the Israelites, are not exempt from death due to rebellion. The New Testament is consistent with the Old Testament in giving a warning to anyone who turns away from God. The Apostle Paul's warning is specific.

> If you live according to the sinful nature, you will die; but if by
> the Spirit you put to death the misdeeds of the body, you will
> live. (Romans 8:13)
>
> For the wages of sin is death but the gift of God is eternal life
> in Christ Jesus our Lord. (Romans 6:23)

These words of warning, the Apostle Paul wrote to those who have already been saved, believing in Jesus and accepting Him as Lord and Savior. Yes, even those who have been justified continue to live under the constant threat of the deadly power of sin. The Apostle Peter writes about those who have fallen away from the truth.

> It would have been better for them not to have known the way
> of righteousness than to have known it and then to turn their
> backs on the sacred command that was passed on to them. (2
> Peter 2:21)

The offer of life or death is in effect for us as well. Repentance changes one's position from being under a curse to being under a blessing. Widespread is the belief that being a victim of violence, betrayal, or deception can justify vengeance, anger, or hatred toward the perpetrator. Such responses are "natural" but sinful. They are the fruit of the old flesh. They are a trap of the enemy to ensnare the believer. Sin is sin under any circumstances, and righteousness is righteousness under all conditions. The practice of one or the other brings death or life, respectively. Like the Israelites, we must choose life over death.

How do we, then, overcome the traps of the enemy? The Holy Church has issued an eternal edict: Confess, repent, forgive, crucify the sinful practices of the flesh, wash in the blood of Jesus spilled on the cross, and fill up with the Holy Spirit. These are part of the holy sacraments of the Church. For the victim, the act of forgiveness might seem impossible, but from heaven's perspective, nothing is impossible for God (Luke 1:37). Faith in Jesus the Messiah is the answer. He gives us the capacity to meet the righteous requirements of the Law through the Spirit of the Living God who dwells in us. The Law cannot impart life, and righteousness does not come through the Law; rather, the Law sets the criteria for determining righteous or sinful living. Just as the curses and the blessings are embedded in the Law, so is the promise of the indwelling of the Holy Spirit in the heart of the believer. For the Spirit-filled Christian, the born-from-above individual, the promise of the Lord is fulfilled.

I will put my law in their minds and write it on their hearts.
(Jeremiah 31:33b)

We have been given a new nature through which sin shall not be our master, because we are not under the law, but under grace (Romans 6:14). But consider an even greater advantage: You have been given fullness in Christ (Colossians 2:10), which is His righteousness and holiness. The recapitulation is straightforward: On the divine judgment scales of life and death, our ability to keep the Law weighs heavily on God's side. It is God who imparts in us His righteousness. Only through Him can we acquire the ability to fulfill the righteous requirements of His Law and live under blessing, not curse. We cannot do this on our own. The Apostle Paul writes about his experience with both conditions, operating under the Law and under God's grace. Being a Pharisee, a highly educated teacher of the Law, the Apostle Paul admits: I found that the very commandment that was intended to bring life actually brought death (Romans 7:10).

The Apostle Paul concluded that no human effort to comply with the Law could genuinely satisfy the requirements of the Law. Humans would always fall short when striving to achieve righteousness on their own. God sees our self-righteous acts as "filthy rags" (Isaiah 64:6). But in Jesus, our position is changed. Through Him, the indwelling power of God enables us to live according to the righteous requirements of the Law. Through Christ Jesus, the law of the Spirit of life set us free from the law of sin and death (Romans 8:2).

If you are saved, born again by the Spirit of God, you have already satisfied all conditions for complete healing from any traumatic experience. You possess the divine tool for healing from pain—His righteousness imparted in you. Commit daily to the spiritual disciplines of prayer, confession, repentance, forgiveness, eucharist, death, and resurrection in Christ Jesus for sanctification and transformation into the image of Christ. These are the holy sacraments of the Church.

EHAD with GOD

REFLECTION—Week Three

Reflection 1: Give Him Five (5 minutes)—the daily practice of God's presence (see description on pages 41 and 63, under "Deep calls to deep" section)

Reflection 2: Daily confession and repentance in prayer to Christ, our high priest; crucify the flesh, wash with the blood, fill with the Holy Spirit (page 13)

Reflection 3: Pray the words of Psalm 121

Reflection 4: The Story of Travis

Psalm 121

Task: Pray the words of Psalm 121. Let this be your song of ascent.

> I lift up my eyes to the hills—where does my help come from? My help comes from the LORD, the Maker of heaven and earth. He will not let your foot slip—he who watches over you will not slumber; indeed, he who watches over Israel will neither slumber nor sleep.
>
> The LORD watches over you— the LORD is your shade at your right hand; the sun will not harm you by day, nor the moon by night. The LORD will keep you from all harm—he will watch over your life; the LORD will watch over your coming and going both now and forevermore. (Psalms 121)

This psalm is God's Word for you, a reminder that you are never alone on the narrow road. As you call upon Jesus' name, ask Him to come near you, to stand by your side, and walk alongside you. Do you hear Him calling you to step up on the narrow road towards your healing? Yes, God is calling you to get out of the slimy pit and walk towards Him! You have no strength to do it? Perhaps you have no desire either, or you just don't care anymore. Your efforts to get out of the pit have all proved worthless. You have tried hard and have failed over and over again. After so many attempts, you are still in the pit, alone in the dark, alone in the cold, crushed in your misery. You have walked broken through life for so long that it has become your "natural" state of existence. You have come to believe that there is no other state of heart besides being trapped in the slimy pit of sadness and pain.

Maybe you did try hard, but your quest for happiness and peace only confirmed your dreadful fears of being hopelessly lost in the maze of endless, unhappy days. Your spirit is starving for love; your soul is longing for rest; your body is aching for a soothing touch. Your failures to break free from pain and misery have only made you more acutely aware of your deepening needs and increasing wants. Maybe you are at the point where the emptiness inside has turned into despair. And there you are—a prisoner to pain and misery.

Listen! Right where you are, at the bottom of the pit. Just listen and consider something else: Things will change for you now; the gloom will be shaken off. Listen! It is not I who says this; your God calls you to listen.

Cheer up! On your feet! He's calling you. (Mark 10:49)

See, God is calling you! He calls your name. Do you hear His voice? Do you feel His breath of life breathed fresh on you? Would you say "Yes" to your God, who in His steadfast love has come to journey on the narrow road with you?

Still the cries of your heart, quiet your soul, and listen! God has spoken to you! "Yes," you say, "but I can't get out of the pit. I can't walk towards God. It is hard for me to lift my head, much less move my feet. It is hard. It is impossible!" Of course, it is hard. It indeed feels impossible. Pain paralyzes, and sorrow stiffens the ability to move. Consuming self-pity binds with cords of helplessness, and deep sadness wraps its nets of utter destitution. Despair imprisons. You are right. From the trappings of this captivity, everything seems impossible. Listen again! While you are unable to move, you can still listen. Tone down and tune up to the voice of God.

> Be still and know that I am God. (Psalm 46:10)

> Fear not, for I have redeemed you; I have summoned you by name; you are mine. (Isaiah 43:1b)

Consider His call and come humbly before Him. Soon, you will find yourself strengthened on the road to freedom.

Note: When you find yourself overwhelmed by sorrow, when emotions are rampaging, and feelings override reason, consider this strategy:

GO WITH THE MOTION, NOT WITH THE EMOTION

Go with the motion of the Cross, described in session one (page 13), with the prayers provided. Be honest, firmly desiring to do what is right in the eyes of God. Don't trust emotions. The heart is deceitful above all things and beyond cure (Jeremiah 17:9). Instead, employ the strategy of simple faith: The believer lives by faith (Habakkuk 2:4). Take this step with complete confidence that the Scripture is truthful and the teachings lead to divine healing. Remember, the Lord knows your state of being "poor in spirit " (Matthew 5:3). His promise is worthy:

> Blessed are the poor in spirit, for theirs is the Kingdom of heaven. (Matthew 5:3)

Jesus will enable you to follow Him. This is precisely what the prayer from the pit will be: To ask Him to give you strength to still your heart so you can hear His voice and follow Him.

Prayer

Lord Jesus, I call to You from the bottom of the pit. Holy Spirit, I invite You to come and minister to me. Let Your healing presence penetrate the deepest caverns of my heart to those places that have never been touched. Lord, I am broken inside and hurting. Darkness and pain have been my only companions for a long time. All my heart feels is pain. All my eyes see is darkness. Your light seems nonexistent. I have forgotten the sweet taste of Your peace. My days are robbed of joy and happiness. I have been held prisoner to despair for a long time. Misery is my bed. Darkness is my cover. In faith, Lord, I call forth Your light to push the darkness that has imprisoned me for so long. I need Your grace to bring my aching soul to stillness. I need Your mercy, Father, to silence the cries of my heart. Quiet my soul so I can be more attentive to Your voice. Still my heart, Lord, make it sensitive to Your presence. Soothe the wounds of my broken spirit. Bring Your light into my darkness. Restore the peace inside. Tune my spirit to Your Spirit so I can hear Your voice and follow You. In Jesus' holy name, I pray. Amen!

Allow yourself time to soak in the presence of the Holy Spirit. You may need to repeat the prayer a few times so your mind's petition comes into agreement with the needs of your heart, because the steps ahead require the unity of both.

Are you ready to approach Jesus as never before? Are you ready to embark on a transforming journey on the narrow road to the Kingdom of heaven? The desired transformation will be a spiritual one: EHAD with God. Your despised state of misery will be replaced with the much-desired state of peace. Come and take the gift from heaven for the cure of your heart. It has been available ever since Jesus declared it two thousand years ago.

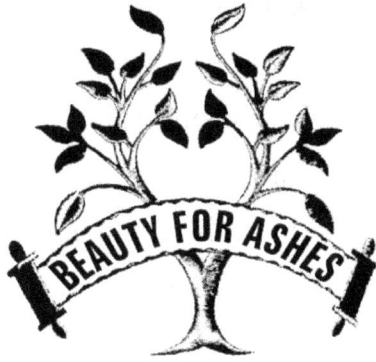

SESSION FOUR

SALVATION AND SANCTIFICATION

Upon salvation, we enter the Kingdom of God with heavy baggage from our wretched lives. Some come merely scratched, some bruised, and still others come stabbed, bleeding to death. This is because we live in a fallen, unredeemed world. We, as a part of this world, are all caught up in a vicious cycle of sin and death: When sin is committed, the divine retribution for punishment is death. A trespass committed in the physical realm triggers deadly consequences in the spiritual realm. Spiritual death leads to more sin. More sin gives evil the right to expand its territory, solidifying the Devil's foothold in the human heart (Ephesians 4:27). Because evil acquires more access to reign in the heart, more laws are broken. More broken laws lead to more evil deeds, thoughts, and desires. This vicious cycle has been in effect in our world since sin entered it. This vicious cycle affects the believer too, unless, through Jesus, we attain His righteousness and break free from the cycle of sin and death (James 1:15). *EHAD with GOD* is the way to freedom.

The brokenness of the world is the cause and the consequence of our wounding and pain. We are broken by the wickedness of a broken world. We cause others pain because of our own brokenness. An innocent soul becomes ill when subjected to the wickedness roaming impetuously throughout the world. No one is insured against emotional pain. When experienced in excess, emotional pain shrivels the soul, causing it to withdraw from the light of life and to huddle in darkness. If the wounds don't heal, the soul sinks to such depths that this painful condition itself becomes a hindrance to the new way of life the believer has in Jesus. But the Scripture tells us there is a way to break the vicious cycle of evil through Christ crucified.

> He was pierced for our transgressions, He was crushed for our
> iniquities; the punishment that brought us peace was upon
> Him, and by His wounds we are healed. (Isaiah 53:5)

We cannot cure the entire world from the consequences of sin, but we can cure ourselves. Then, our healing affects the world around us, and we become instruments for the healing of others. We become agents of good, not evil. The vicious cycle of sin and death in our lives and the world around us is broken! And this wonderful "destruction" happens through Jesus' peace in a healed heart! Jesus left His peace with us (John 14:27). It takes some time for this wonderful transformation to happen, but once the Lord starts it, He brings it to completion. This is the process through which we are infused with the righteous attributes of Christ as we simultaneously remove everything incompatible with the Kingdom of God. The Lord God accepts us just as we are, broken and imperfect. He begins to cleanse and mold us until we conform, in mind and heart, after His initial design: His holiness and righteousness become mirrored in us (1 Corinthians 1:30). This is **sanctification**. Faith in Jesus resurrects the human spirit, which was dead, a condition we all inherited since the Fall. This is **salvation**.

> He was delivered over to death for our sins and was raised to
> life for our justification. (Romans 4:25)

On the Cross, a magnificent spiritual transaction happens: The transfer of guilt from a sinner to Jesus. In the Old Testament, the guilt was transferred by laying hands on the head of the animal. It was a substitute offering, which God accepted on people's behalf to make atonement for them (Leviticus 1:4; Leviticus 3:2, 4:4, 8, 13, 24, 29, 33). Transferring the sin on the animal was a way to identify with it as it was sacrificed to atone for the person's sins. The spiritual act of accepting Jesus as a personal savior serves the same purpose. On the Cross, the sins of the world were placed on Him.

> The Lord has laid on him the iniquity of us all. (Isaiah 53:6)

> He is the atoning sacrifice for our sins, and not only for ours but also for the sins of the whole world. (1 John 2:2)

The death of Jesus on the Cross is a substitutional offering. It is **salvation** for all who accept it. On the Cross of Jesus, another magnificent spiritual transaction happened: The transfer of the holiness of Christ.

> ... we have been made holy through the sacrifice of the body of Jesus Christ once for all." (Hebrews 10:10)

In the Old Testament, the sacrifice offered on a consecrated altar was considered holy; everything it touched, its flesh or blood, was considered consecrated and made holy also (Leviticus 6:27). The sacrifice became holy because the altar was holy. Moses received special instructions on how to consecrate the altar of the Tabernacle. It required a seven-day ritual involving anointing with oil and the application of the sacrificial blood of a bull and a ram (Exodus 29). Their blood was sprinkled on the horns and the base of the altar, thus making it holy. Only after its consecration, the altar became holy. The holiness of Jesus consecrated the Cross, made it holy. Everyone who accepts His sacrifice for their sins comes in contact with the Cross, the altar, and its holiness is transferred to the believer. This is **sanctification**.

At the moment of salvation, we are like newborn babies, craving pure spiritual milk so that we may grow up in our salvation (1 Peter 2:2). However, many of His saved people never mature spiritually, ready to digest solid food. Healing the heart from pain requires a solid food spiritual diet.

Continuing to live in sin after accepting Christ is profaning His holiness that was transferred to the person upon salvation. This is defilement. It is a spiritual condition that impedes maturity in the faith and the relationship with the Lord. The state of emotional misery is a consequence of spiritual immaturity. If the sins are not confessed and forgiven, they become a stronghold in a person's life, giving a "foothold" to the Devil to "steal, kill, and destroy" (John 10:10). The condition of the person continues to deteriorate.

Upon salvation, the restoration of humanity back to God's original design has just begun. That was the moment when the curtain in the Holy of Holies was torn in two (Luke 23:45; Matthew 27:51), allowing the redeemed to approach God's presence as never before. Many believers, however, have remained at the entrance of the Kingdom, at the ripped curtain, never entering the Holy of Holies, having communion with God. Healing from pain happens in the Holy of Holies, where God dwells. The Holy of Holies of the ancient Temple is the believer's heart today.

> Don't you know that you yourselves are God's Temple and that
> God's Spirit lives in you? (1 Corinthians 3:16)

In ancient times, the glory of God resided in the Holy of Holies, in the ancient Temple. And if the Temple is the human heart today, then the same glory resides in the heart of every believer. There is a difference between the glory of God radiating from Moses and the glory of God radiating within a believer's heart. When Moses came down from Mount Sinai with the two tablets of the covenant, his face was radiant because he had spoken with the Lord. The glory of God was imprinted on Moses. He had to put a veil over his face when meeting with the people (Ex 34:29-35). Moses' radiant glow faded with time. For today's believers, the glory of God radiates from within without fading.

> We, who with unveiled faces all reflect the Lord's glory, are
> being transformed into his likeness with ever-increasing glory,

which comes from the Lord, who is the Spirit. (2 Corinthians 3:18)

In this "ever-increasing glory," there is no pain and misery because the sanctification and the transformation into the image of Christ have happened. And if Christ indeed dwells in you, then His presence is peace, not pain. Healing is not a static position of waiting and wailing but the action of approaching and actively seeking the One who holds the power to exchange the ashes of our misery with a crown of beauty (Isaiah 61:3).

Similarly, as it is with the call for **salvation**, in which one must personally confess and receive forgiveness of sin, so it is with the call for **sanctification**: One must take the cross daily and follow Jesus (Luke 9:23). Salvation is a gift of God (Ephesians 2:8), but once received, says the Apostle Paul, we must work out our salvation with fear and trembling (Philippians 2:12). Apostle James encourages to seek God.

Come near to God and He will come near to you. (James 4:8a)

But he also tells us how to approach God.

Wash your hands, you sinners, and purify your hearts, you double-minded. (James 4:8b)

The psalmist affirms the criteria for entering God's presence:

Who may ascend the hill of the LORD? Who may stand in his holy place? He who has clean hands and a pure heart, who does not lift up his soul to an idol or swear by what is false. He will receive blessing from the LORD and vindication from God his Savior. (Psalms 24:3,4)

Upon salvation, we are justified, but only when we sanctify ourselves may we ascend to the hill of the Lord with clean hands and a pure heart. The discussion that follows will explain how the requirements for cleansing of today's believers mirror the requirements for cleansing in ancient Israel. As the ancient worshipers had a cleansing ritual before approaching God, the same is expected from today's believers; we must also satisfy the requirements for purity when approaching God. Everything else is hypocrisy. People may not see it, but God does, and instead of a blessing, we incur judgment (1 Corinthians 11:23-29).

Purification and Sanctification in the Old Testament

The blood of Jesus spilled on the Cross has a crucial significance in the healing from traumatic events. To understand the role of the blood in the healing process, we have to look at its importance in the Old and the New Testaments.

The Old Testament's sacrificial system was set on the shedding of animal blood. Entering into God's presence in the Holy of Holies required conformity of heart after God's nature; one must be pure and holy, like God, to enter His presence.

> Be holy because I, the LORD your God, am holy! (Leviticus 19:2)

This is God's requirement for humankind. The call for purification and sanctification recurs throughout the Old Testament. No one could approach God without first being cleansed from the defilement of sin. As the Law is irrevocable, so is the condition for one's purification for entering God's presence because God has spoken both. In the same way, we, the believers in Christ, are warned that no one can enter the Kingdom of God unless one is cleansed from all impurities (Colossians 3:5).

> Put to death, therefore, whatever belongs to your earthly nature: sexual immorality, impurity, lust, evil desires and greed, which is idolatry. Because of these, the wrath of God is coming. You used to walk in these ways, in the life you once lived. But now you must rid yourselves of all such things as these: anger, rage, malice, slander, and filthy language from your lips. Do not lie to each other, since you have taken off

your old self with its practices and have put on the new self, which is being renewed in knowledge in the image of its Creator. (Colossians 3:5-10)

The pages of the Old Testament are "stained" with the blood of sacrificial animals for purification and sanctification. Once a year, on Yom Kippur—the Day of Atonement—only the high priest was to enter the presence of God into the Holy of Holies, where He resided. The Lord God gave thorough instructions to Moses concerning how Aaron, as a high priest, should purify and consecrate himself to enter God's presence and not die. God warned Aaron not to come into the Most Holy Place behind the curtain whenever he chose, or else he would die, because God appears in the cloud over the atonement cover (Leviticus 16:2). The office of the high priest did not give Aaron the right to come into the Holy of Holies; only his condition of purity permitted his entrance. If Aaron was not ritually cleansed when entering the presence of God, he would have died.

In accordance with the requirements for purity, the path from the altar to the Holy of Holies, the place for meeting with God, was sprinkled with blood—from the horns of the altar to its base (Exodus 29:12). The high priest also had to be sprinkled with blood—from the lobes of the right ear to the big toe of the right foot (Exodus 29:20). These repulsive instructions better fit the description of a butcher shop or a crime scene, not a process of purification. According to our human standards, the sight of sticky, smelly, dried blood is nothing but unclean, but from God's perspective, the outside appearance is not a concern. It is the inside of us that God wants to cleanse from the defilement of sin. Only the blood of a perfect sacrificial animal could purify the soul. According to the just retributions of God's Law, "the soul who sins is the one who will die" (Ezekiel 18:4, 20), but according to God's love, He redeems that life through another life, that of an animal.

For the life of a creature is in the blood, and I have given it to you to make atonement for yourselves on the altar; it is the blood that makes atonement for one's life. (Leviticus 17:11)

Purification and Sanctification in the New Testament

The mystery of the Cross is a pattern embedded in the Old Testament sacrificial system—death for life. The required burnt offering was an atonement offering. According to this understanding, Apostle Paul calls the believers to offer themselves as a living sacrifice on the altar of Jesus as true and proper worship. The Cross is our altar.

Therefore, I urge you, brothers and sisters, in view of God's mercy, to offer your bodies as a living sacrifice, holy and pleasing to God—this is your true and proper worship. (Romans 12:1)

This is the spiritual act of offering ourselves as a burnt offering, a pleasing aroma to the Lord (Leviticus 1:9). Burning the old nature on the altar of God is equivalent to "take your cross daily" (Luke 9:23). It is a spiritual act of putting to death whatever belongs to the earthly nature (Colossians 3:5). It is an act of faith to move from death to life.

For if you live according to the flesh, you will die; but if by the Spirit you put to death the misdeeds of the body, you will live. (Romans 8:13)

The believers in Christ don't depend on the blood of sacrificial animals for cleansing. The blood of Jesus shed on the cross satisfied all requirements for purification. He is God's holy Lamb, and His blood atoned for the sins of the world, once and for all. It is a spiritual Law! The Giver of Life became the Redeemer of life. No one else but God Himself paid the ransom for our sins. No one else is pure and perfect to take the place of a perfect sacrificial animal. He, the holy and the righteous One, took our punishment, and we, the sinners, were set free. Incomprehensible love! How much higher are His ways than our ways! The Prophet Isaiah prophesied the redemptive mission of God as Jesus the Messiah.

> The LORD looked and was displeased that there was no justice. He saw that there was no one, he was appalled that there was no one to intervene; so his own arm worked salvation for him, and his own righteousness sustained him. He put on righteousness as his breastplate, and the helmet of salvation on his head; he put on the garments of vengeance and wrapped himself in zeal as in a cloak. (Isaiah 59:15-17)

Jesus is referred to in the Scripture as the Lamb of God. The Old Testament required a perfect young, male animal without blemish (Exodus 12:05). Jesus lived a sinless life and satisfied the requirements, taking the place of the sacrificial lamb. He is our Passover lamb that has been sacrificed (1 Corinthians 5:7). When John the Baptist first saw Jesus, he referred to Him as the Lamb of God.

> Look! The Lamb of God who takes away the sin of the world!
> (John 1:36)

On the island of Patmos, Apostle John received visions in an end-time context. He referred to Jesus as "a Lamb, looking as if it had been slain" (Revelation 5:6). Later, he also decrees that the believers will be victorious in defeating the Devil "by the blood of the Lamb" (Revelation 12:5) and assures the believers under persecution of the Lamb's ultimate authority over eternal life and death.

> All inhabitants of the earth will worship the beast—all whose names have not been written in the book of life, belonging to the Lamb that was slain from the creation of the world. (Revelation 13:8)

Apostle John also gives us a glimpse of eternity in the New Jerusalem,

> I did not see a temple in the city, because the Lord God Almighty and the Lamb are its Temple. (Revelation 21:22)

At the end of his testimony, Apostle John describes the ultimate EHAD, where God and humanity regain their fellowship as designed in the Garden of Eden. The New Jerusalem is the old Garden of Eden! This is the "new thing" which God foretold through the Prophet Isaiah long ago:

> Forget the former things; do not dwell on the past. See, I am doing a new thing! Now it springs up; do you not perceive it? (Isaiah 43:18-19)

The Way of Holiness

In the book of Acts, the followers of Jesus are called the followers of the Way (Acts 9:2; 19:9, 23; 22:4; 24:14,22). The name appears to reference Jesus' teaching.

> I am the way and the truth and the life. No one comes to the Father except through me. (John 14:6)

The narrow road is the Way on which Christ's followers attain Christ's holiness. It is the road of **sanctification**. In His last prayer in Gethsemane, Jesus prayed for the disciples and those who will believe in Him through their message (John 17:20). He asked for complete unity of God and believers, that they become EHAD (John 17:22) just as God the Father and Jesus are EHAD (John 17:23). Jesus prayed for oneness of the believers with God as supposed oneness with the world. The distinction is in the state of heart of a believer in which Jesus Himself dwells (John 17:26). This is the essence of becoming EHAD with God. This is the Way of Holiness. The transformation into the image of Christ transforms the common into holy.

Holy Yet Corrupt—Cognitive Dissonance

The redemptive power of the blood of Jesus washes us pure, but the corrupt condition of the soul continues to bring constant defilement from the fallen world, the flesh, and the enemy. The Lord God has not waived the requirement for purity to enter into His presence. Like our spiritual ancestors, we must purify and sanctify ourselves to approach God. The Apostle Paul repeatedly pleaded with the believers to listen to his appeal for perfection (1 Corinthians 13:11). We are called to be holy (1 Corinthians 1:3; 1 Peter 1:16) because He chose us in Him before the creation of the world to be holy and blameless in His sight (Ephesians 1:4). Jesus instructed us to be perfect because our heavenly Father is perfect (Matthew 5:48). Our Lord would never ask anything from His children without providing the means to accomplish it. The blood and the cross of Jesus are the believers' means for satisfying God's requirements for purity and holiness. The cross heals the corrupt state of the heart, and the blood washes it pure. This is a continuous process of death and resurrection through which the old nature of flesh is replaced with the righteousness of Christ. We enter God's presence without the threat of death as Aaron did but with the promise of transformation into His glory.

The Apostle Paul calls this transformation into holiness and perfection a "mystery, which is Christ in you, the hope of glory" (Colossians 1:27). Holiness is an intrinsic characteristic of God's very nature. Humankind can achieve holiness only by being transformed into the image of Christ, the Lord God Himself. This is the process of becoming EHAD with Jesus. He spoke of this transformation, saying,

> On that day, you will realize that I am in my Father and you
> are in me, and I am in you. (John 14:20)

When, in your own life, "that day" comes to pass, and you become aware of being EHAD with Christ, then great will your assurance be, knowing that you are walking on the road of holiness. It is no longer you who exhibits godly attributes but Christ living in you (Galatians 2:20); His holiness and His perfection (not yours) are manifesting in your life. King David wrote about the requirements for entering the presence of the Lord.

> LORD, who may dwell in your sanctuary? Who may live on
> your holy hill? He whose walk is blameless and who does what

is righteous, who speaks the truth from his heart and has no slander on his tongue, who does his neighbor no wrong and casts no slur on his fellowman, who despises a vile man but honors those who fear the LORD, who keeps his oath even when it hurts, who lends his money without usury and does not accept a bribe against the innocent. He who does these things will never be shaken. (Psalms 15:1-5)

When we come to the Father purified, sanctified, and transformed, our oneness with Him as designed at the beginning of time is restored. Through the redemption of the soul (**salvation**) and its healing (**sanctification**), God's requirements for becoming EHAD with Him are satisfied.

The cure from traumatic experiences proceeds from our restoration to the initial divine design, which mirrored God's likeness and image (Colossians 3:10). Through Jesus, we regain our new self, created to be like God in true righteousness and holiness (Ephesians 4:24). We are given fullness in Christ (Colossians 2:10). We have been restored to our uncorrupted design, back to the Garden of Eden design.

The process of attaining the fullness in Christ starts with the justification of sin (**salvation**); it proceeds with cleansing from defilement (**sanctification**); it culminates with a transformation into the likeness of Christ. At that point, we have become EHAD with Christ.

Oaks of Righteousness

True transformation occurs when there is nothing more to be taken from the old nature of flesh but more to be added to the new nature one gains in Christ. After removing sin and impurities, we must replace them with the righteous attributes of Christ. Jesus made this process of purification and sanctification possible to all who accept His free sacrificial gift. Through Christ, believers now have the potential to become holy and perfect as God Himself. Jesus plants the seed of righteousness in the believer's heart to grow into a mighty tree rooted in eternal life. We are called to become oaks of righteousness, a planting of the Lord for the display of His splendor (Isaiah 61:3).

What a call! Whoever looks at a believer in Christ should see God's splendor and glory! Now consider asking yourself, "Am I, as a believer in Jesus, a true display of God's splendor?" What would the answer be?

Question: What are the things that prevent me from being a channel for the display of God's splendor? Write down practices and behaviors incompatible with the Kingdom of God.

_____

_____

_____

_____

_____

_____

_____

Defilement From Sin

The list that proceeds from such examination pins down the areas in our lives that are still governed by the old, sinful nature of flesh (Romans 7:18). These are the deepest corners of the heart that have not been crucified with Jesus yet. These are the practices of the flesh that have not been renounced and hauled to the cross. These are the sinful thoughts, desires, and passions that function as an open door for demonic entities to gain a foothold in the hearts of believers. These are the strongholds of evil devouring us within our flesh.

Examine yourself to determine what grieves the Spirit of God. Defilement proceeds from the continuous presence of sin in the heart of the believer: The old patterns of behavior, attitudes of heart, and thoughts that have not yet conformed with the Kingdom of God. The Apostle Paul identifies the practice of sin as being "at work in the members of my body" (Romans 7:23). He honestly speaks about his struggles:

> For I have the desire to do what is good, but I cannot carry it out. For what I do is not the good I want to do; no, the evil I do not want to do—this I keep on doing. Now if I do what I do not want to do, it is no longer I who do it, but it is the sin in me that does it. (Romans 7:18-20)

You may identify with Apostle Paul's struggles, groaning in frustration, losing hope, and plunging in despair over the overwhelming power of sin. Your struggle is nothing new under the sun (Ecclesiastes 1:9). This struggle happens daily on the narrow road toward eternity with God, even with Jesus next to us. This is the ever-present struggle with our thinking structures, distorted emotions, and corrupt habits of our old nature that lead to defilement. The process of spiritual maturity entails this grueling struggle with sin. We have been called to endure it ever since sin afflicted humankind: Sin is crouching at your door; it desires to have you, but you must master it (Genesis 4:7b).

The reward of enduring these struggles is worthy. To those who overcome sin is the promise of eternal life in the Kingdom of God (Revelation 2:7,11,17,26; 3:5,12,21). How are we to endure? How are we to overcome? The Bible tells us that a true believer should exhibit the fruit of the Spirit: Love, joy, peace, patience, kindness, goodness, faithfulness, gentleness, and self-control (Galatians 5:22-23); not pain, fear, loneliness, desperation, anger, hatred, or despair. The latter are manifestations of the old flesh, and they must be put to death on the cross.

> Those who belong to Christ Jesus have crucified the sinful nature with its passions and desires. (Galatians 5:24)

Those who belong to Christ have risen to new life (Romans 6:4). As we die with Christ to the pains of the old nature, we also rise with Him to the joy of becoming new creations. When we crucify our old "self" with Christ, it is no longer we who live, but it is Christ who lives in us (Galatians 2:20); and if

Christ lives in us, it is not our righteousness but His righteousness that we have, not our joy but His joy, not our peace but His peace. Thus, the presence of Christ pushes out despair and pain. In Him, we are a new creation; the old has gone, (along with suffering and pain), the new has come (2 Corinthians 5:17). The more one attains Christ's nature, the stronger one becomes at resisting and overcoming sin and emotional pain. Through the cross, the pain indeed is destined to complete annihilation.

The reality, however, is different. Many redeemed people continue to be overwhelmed by unbearable pain. Pain is a consequence of being alienated from God because of: 1) sin or 2) immaturity in growing in the image of Christ and becoming EHAD with Him. The second reason presupposes the first, and the first reason assures that the second happens, e.g., if we are spiritually immature, we are bound to sin, and if we sin, we cannot mature spiritually. The usual culprit of this stagnation in spiritual growth is unredemptive emotional pain.

Defilement From Unredemptive Emotional Pain

Apostle Paul speaks of two kinds of sorrows: Godly and worldly.

Godly sorrow brings repentance that leads to salvation and leaves no regret, but worldly sorrow brings death. (2 Corinthians 7:10)

Worldly sorrow is self-destructive. Harboring anger, hatred, resentment, bitterness, unforgiveness, and animosity toward an offender only harms the victim, not the perpetrator. These are practices of the flesh that constitute unredemptive emotional pain. They seem the most "natural" response of a trauma victim toward the offender, but they cause defilement of the victim. Hypothetically, if the offender repents from the wrongdoing, God grants forgiveness, even if the victim is not willing to forgive. In this situation, the perpetrator is in the right standing with God, while the victim is guilty of harboring anger and the alike attitudes of the heart. They cause alienation from

God and a failure to grow in the image of Christ, becoming EHAD with Him. We are warned to be aware of such bitter root defilement:

> See to it that no one falls short of the grace of God and that no bitter root grows up to cause trouble and defile many. (Hebrews 12:15)

Godly sorrow is the overwhelming regret the believer experiences from grieving the Lord. It is a righteous response to acknowledging wrongdoing, humbling oneself with a penitent heart. Jesus refers to this state of being poor in spirit that grants entrance to the Kingdom of heaven (Matthew 5:3). This godly sorrow produces a harvest of sustained spiritual growth.

> This godly sorrow has produced in you: what earnestness, what eagerness to clear yourselves, what indignation, what alarm, what longing, what concern, what readiness to see justice done. (2 Corinthians 7:11)

Exhibiting worldly sorrow drifts the believer from the narrow road. Restoration begins with a penitent heart. We must confess and repent when we willingly or unwillingly stray from the narrow road due to worldly sorrow. There is no condemnation for those in Christ Jesus (Romans 8:1). Confession and repentance restore the believer to a rightful position with God. Godly sorrow is an attitude of repentance, an experience from which we must learn and grow, never to repeat the offense. Otherwise, we are likened to a dog that returns to its own vomit, and a fool that repeats his folly (Proverbs 26:11). Examples of godly sorrow are the presence of genuine remorse after gossiping, stealing, manipulating, abusing, neglecting God and His Word, not attending church services, disrespecting parents, coveting, adultery, anger, hatred, bitterness, resentment, judgmental attitudes, guilt, self-condemnation, etc. Even perpetrators of rape, murder, incest, and violence find redemption when they approach God with godly sorrow. This is a spiritual Law. If God forgives the offender, should the victim forgive too?

God's Kingdom is not anger, unforgiveness, or bitterness but peace, joy, and love. The believer must choose the path of godly sorrow, becoming aware of the destructive consequences of vengeance, rejecting them, and embracing forgiveness and mercy instead. Only then does the victim become a victor, and only then will healing from the trauma begin. Vengeance belongs to God.

It is mine to avenge; I will repay, says the LORD.

(Deuteronomy 32:35)

Unredemptive emotional pain is an illness of the soul (heart) that prevents the believer from experiencing the fullness of life in Christ. It may proceed from wounds suffered before or after salvation. Both conditions are hallmarked by captivity foreign to the Kingdom of God.

God designed us to accept and react to information received through our senses (smell, touch, taste, hearing, sight), with which we explore and survive in the physical environment. Physical pain alerts us to danger to our physical existence. We immediately flee from the source of pain or take steps to alleviate it. Just as physical pain indicates an affliction against the body, so is emotional pain indicative of an affliction within the soul. When we touch a hot surface, we immediately escape the source of danger. We may get a blister, but we don't wait to see the skin engulfed in flames. The response to emotional pain, though, is different. It accumulates undetected, piling ache upon ache, usually over prolonged periods. Emotional and verbal abuse is a trauma that inflicts "blister" after "blister" upon the sufferer, but neither the abuser nor the victim is aware of its deadly effect. Left untreated, the blistered wounds could easily become inflamed.

In most cases, the victim is tied to the abuser through family or life circumstances, which ensures inflammation that creates open, bleeding, festering wounds. No one neglects seeking medical attention for a physical wound, but a festering emotional wound is often left untreated and ultimately ignored. Also, neglect is the source of the wound. Unaware of the damaging long-term effects of emotional wounding, we are hopelessly ill-equipped to defend ourselves or those dependent on us (our children) from the causes of hurt. The irony of any abusive situation lies in the depth of emotional dependency upon and the feelings invested in the relationship: The more we love those who inflict pain on us, the more we hurt. Satan has turned the source of our love and nurture into a source of pain and death. This kind of death, however, comes unseen; its origin is hard to detect. While physical abuse is easy to prosecute based on visible evidence, emotional abuse is difficult to prove.

Emotional wounding is like a thick shroud enveloping the heart or an iron cage that holds it captive. It is a condition of indefinite imprisonment to pain and suffering. If the condition is not treated, the soul sinks further into the miry depths of despair. At some indeterminate point, suffering becomes so excruciating that death seems a desired escape. Depression and suicidal ideation are common manifestations at this stage, which is indicative of the severity of the affliction.

When wounded individuals enter the Kingdom of God, the presence of the Holy Spirit penetrates the core of their beings, searching, cleansing, and healing. This sanctifying work of the Holy Spirit brings salvation and begins the healing of the human soul. He restores our spiritual sight and hearing. We are in a state of EHAD with God.

Healing, however, does not happen immediately upon entering the Kingdom of God. Even though salvation and healing are like the head and the tail of a coin, each takes a different time to be engraved onto the heart. While **salvation** is an immediate occurrence (upon confession of sin and acceptance of Christ), healing is the process of **sanctification** and transformation into the image of Christ. Salvation is immediate, and at that point, we are saved positionally. Salvation is also simultaneously progressive, and it happens daily on our walk on the narrow road. The Scripture tells us that to those being saved (1 Corinthians 1:18), sanctification is the means to our ongoing salvation, accomplished through the sanctifying work of the Holy Spirit and belief in the truth (2 Thessalonians 2:13). This is the process of regaining the fullness of God as designed at the beginning of time. The knowledge of healing through sanctification and transformation in the image of Christ is an immensely valuable asset in the hands of every believer to counteract the pangs of unredemptive emotional pain.

There is a difference between the status of the emotional wounding of a nonbeliever and a believer in Christ. While they both are captive to the same prison of emotional pain, the captivity of the believer is only subjective. Upon salvation, despite the "first love" excitement, the believer's heart may remain a prison tower due to prior traumatic experiences. However, the land on which that tower stands has now been redeemed. God's law of redemption postulates that all gates of the dungeon must be open wide and the subjects set free. Instead of leaping out to freedom, many believers remain bound, tightly fastened with cords of pain, with no chance for the healing presence of the Spirit of God to enter and heal. Under the veil of emotional pain, these believers don't realize they have been set free, even free from pain. They continue to wail and mourn their miserable condition, loudly begging for help, without understanding that the same law of redemption that opened the prison gates also holds the power to break the chains of captivity to emotional pain. Yes, the same power that redeems the soul from the sting of death also heals the soul from the pangs of emotional pain. Sanctification through Jesus Christ is the way to heal the soul.

> I am the way and the truth and the life. No one comes to the
> Father except through me. (John 14:6)

Coming to the Father is entering through the narrow gate and stepping beyond the ripped curtain of the Holy of Holies, where His presence dwells. There, facing the mercy seat, the redeemed of the Lord find healing.

EHAD with GOD

REFLECTION—Week Four

Reflection 1: Give Him 5—practicing God's presence (pages 41 and 63)

Reflection 2: Daily confession and repentance in prayer to Christ—our high priest; crucify the flesh, wash with the blood, fill with the Holy Spirit (page 13)

Reflection 3: Read Psalm 42 and answer the question below

Reflection 4: The Story of Mia

Psalms 42

As the deer pants for streams of water, so my soul pants for you, O God. My soul thirsts for God, for the living God.

When can I go and meet with God? My tears have been my food day and night, while people say to me all day long, "Where is your God?"

These things I remember as I pour out my soul: how I used to go with the multitude, leading the procession to the house of God, with shouts of joy and thanksgiving among the festive throng. Why are you downcast, O my soul? Why so disturbed within me? Put your hope in God, for I will yet praise him, my Savior and my God.

My soul is downcast within me; therefore, I will remember you from the land of the Jordan, the heights of Hermon—from Mount Mizar.

Deep calls to deep in the roar of your waterfalls; all your waves and breakers have swept over me. By day the LORD directs his love, at night his song is with me—a prayer to the God of my life.

I say to God my Rock, "Why have you forgotten me? Why must I go about mourning, oppressed by the enemy?"

My bones suffer mortal agony as my foes taunt me, saying to me all day long, "Where is your God?" Why are you downcast, O my soul? Why so disturbed within me? Put your hope in God, for I will yet praise him, my Savior and my God.

Question: What would it take for my downcast soul to trust God?

_____

_____

_____

_____

The Story of Mia

Mia was in junior high school when her problems began. She exhibited very low self-esteem. Unpredictable bouts of rage often spout vulgarity, transforming her otherwise unnoticeable demeanor into a paragon of malevolence. She rarely spoke in public and never dared to voice her opinion. Cold indifference toward any academic work ran through her veins. She despised order, skills, excellence, and capability, a bitter reminder of how unattainable these prosperous life goals were for her. She could never be that perfect. She hated anyone who was. Mia was a rebel, angry with the world.

As a young student, she longed to integrate into the larger class community, but she remained "hidden"; she feared others would notice her inadequacy and reject and mock her. This inner conflict triggered her rage. Repeated visits to the counselor's office for numerous fights did nothing to stop her from defying the school's ordinances. She didn't care.

Life had dealt Mia a hard hand. Mia had a horrendous childhood. She was the third of four siblings, living in a slum-like condition in a small town in northern Illinois. Her mother was physically abusive to the point of insanity. It seemed to Mia that she was the only object of her mother's rage. Mia was then just a five-year-old little girl. The physical pain she learned to endure, holding those tears back. Her mother, then, further infuriated, would throw herself at her, screaming, inflicting more pain on her already battered body.

She was eight when her mother left the family, never to return. Mia breathed a sigh of relief for a life without her abuser. The beating stopped, but something more menacing replaced it. Her two brothers began sexually molesting her. The abusive mother stamped Mia's heart with the message that love comes with pain. Her brothers further ingrained in her young mind that the reality of living in pain was the norm, not the exception.

After her mother abandoned the family, her Father went into depression. He began working long hours, drowning his sorrows. The children were left to tend to themselves. Mia shared a bed with her younger sister. Initially, the brothers would come at night for comfort, but very soon, when their baby sister would be asleep, this closeness would turn into a sexual exploration. The sexual abuse continued for many long years. For Mia, this was her brothers' love, but as the years went on, she began dreading the experience. She tried multiple strategies to discourage them from pursuing her, but none were successful. Unmitigated, the daily practice of sexual abuse became the family's "new normal."

It was not until middle school that her troublesome behavioral problems skyrocketed, and she was repeatedly sent to the counselor's office for fighting. On one of these visits, enraged and defiant, she burst out at the counselor, screaming furiously. The accumulated anger towards her brothers found an outlet in the counselor's office. Shouting, she blurted out: "I cannot do this anymore!" Her sexual abuse was no longer a secret. Mia was detained and placed in the foster care system for safety.

Mia loved her brothers and could not shake the guilt of turning them over to the authorities. She also hated the person she had become. She was ravaged by shame, guilt, anger, rage, hatred, animosity, and bitterness. The journey of Mia's healing had just begun.

Task: Take Mia on a healing journey through the road of the cross.

_____
_____
_____
_____
_____

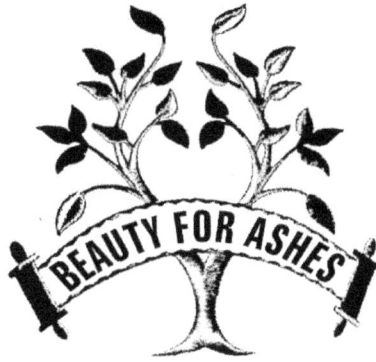

SESSION FIVE

THE POWER OF CONFESSION AND REPENTANCE

A young couple asked pastor Dave for a prayer. The husband was a young minister, and pastor Dave knew the family well. At the set appointment, they came together with their two small children. The day before, pastor Dave inquired of the Lord how to pray for them. "They need to be watered," pastor Dave heard the Lord saying. Water is a sign of the presence of God's Holy Spirit, so pastor Dave understood that he had to center his prayer on inviting the Holy Spirit to minister to them.

That same night, in a dream, the Lord showed pastor Dave, in greater detail, the desperate, water-deprived condition of the family. In his dream, he saw the whole family, the husband, the wife, and their minor children, in what appeared to be an open desert space. Everywhere the eye could see was a dry, arid land with deep cracks splitting the surface. The sun was at its zenith, scourging the ground with unbearable heat. But everyone in the family looked very fresh, especially the wife. She was smiling and talking, completely unaware of the harsh environment. They all were under a deep shade, so deep that pastor Dave could not clearly see the face of the husband, who was just a step behind his wife.

A bald desert mountain was far away on the horizon, as a perfect backdrop to the flat wilderness. On its top, a dark cloud lurked; its ominous presence conveyed an imminent threat, ready to rain down like a flood over the family. That flood had a diabolical quality; it threatened the life of the family. They had to be watered with good water before the threat of the flood swept over them. It was urgent!

At that moment, pastor Dave woke up and began asking the Lord,

"Why are they in the dry?"

"Because their water has been cut off, their cisterns are dry," the Lord answered. "Why was their water cut off? And why are their cisterns dry?" he asked again. "The man knows," the Lord answered.

Then, pastor Dave thought of the shade that covered the family, his mind searching for an explanation. What was the protection over the family that shielded them from the desert scourge? He wondered. It was not a gazebo, for he did not see any structure. A tree with thick branches could give such dense shade, but it was a desert place where no tree could grow. Then he heard the Lord saying, "It is my wing! They are under my wing!" And then he remembered seeing it! Yes, in his dream, he saw the ends of what appeared to be giant feathers. His mind went wild, trying to imagine the size of the wing spread over the entire family that provided such deep shade. The images came with Scripture that gave further direction for prayer.

> How priceless is your unfailing love! Both high and low among men find refuge in the shadow of your wings. They feast on the abundance of your house; you give them drink from your river of delights. For with you is the fountain of life. (Psalm 36:7-8)

Pastor Dave was astonished to see the love and care with which the Lord had shielded the family. In times of trouble, His wing extended over them even though they were neither aware of the extent of danger nor the totality of their protection. But God knew it all, and He sheltered them under His wing because He loved them!

The next day, before the prayer meeting, pastor Dave related the dream to the husband. His face turned pale, and he remained silent. With his head dropped low, he walked away slowly.

Not too long after, pastor Dave noticed with wonder the changes in the young man. His preaching and prayers were no longer dry, an indication that his supplies of living water had been renewed. Whether the turning point of his renewal was before or after the prayer, pastor Dave didn't know, but the Lord knew. Everyone saw clearly displayed in public what the Lord had done in private with this man's heart. This remarkable change from being dry to springing with fountains of living water began with a spirit of repentance. Whatever sin had burdened the man, he faithfully repented and took it to the cross of Jesus. God responded with a renewed supply of living water.

The opposite is also a reality when we often witness the devastating consequences of an unrepentant heart. Words of discernment are frequently met with scorn and mockery. As much as we rejoice in the healing of one, we are deeply saddened by the self-destructive will of the other, and so is the Lord.

The Spirit-to-spirit communication with God requires that we become more like Him. We must conform in the likeness of Christ. The scriptural way of this transformation is repentance from sin and renunciation of wrongdoings. It is not what we do apart from our prayer that changes us, but what God does with us during our prayer when we come with penitent hearts before Him. This is the state of being poor in spirit (Matthew 5:3) that lays the foundations for a new life in Jesus. Then, what God has done in secret in our inner room in prayer (Matthew 6:6), is seen by everyone in the life of that individual for His glory. The first step towards becoming more like Jesus is repentance. Apostle John says,

> If we claim to be without sin, we deceive ourselves, and the
> truth is not in us. (1 John 1:8)

We are urged to look deeper! We are instructed to clean up our lives! We are called to repent! The Israelites lamented and complained to God,

> Our offenses and sins weigh us down, and we are wasting away because of them. How, then, can we live? (Ezekiel 33:10)

The Israelites identified the reason for their suffering, but they did not repent of it. Lord God spoke to the unrepentant house of Israel,

> Turn! Turn from your evil ways! Why will you die, O house of Israel? (Ezekiel 33:11)

The sincere turning away from sin is the act of repentance. The Word from God, delivered through the Prophet Ezekiel, gave the Israelites an understanding of how to end the plague of "wasting away" in sin. They had to turn from evil by repenting and abandoning their sinful practices. What should our response be? Identifying sin alone is not enough to cancel death as retribution for committing it; only repentance from sin can cancel the punishment of death. For the Israelites, this was the turning point from death to life. Not only does the recognition of sin matter to God, but the sincere renunciation by those who practice it. This is the core of the act of repentance. Knowledge of sin does not save; it only convicts of wrongdoing. The power of repentance is in the act of turning away from sin.

> He who conceals his sins does not prosper, but whoever confesses and renounces them finds mercy. (Proverbs 28:13)

An act of repentance unleashes forces in the spiritual realm that operate on the power of God's spoken Word, evoking God's mercy and bringing God's promise for restoration into existence in our lives immediately (Deuteronomy 30:1-10).

Repentance is the turning point of healing. It unleashes forces in the spiritual realm that affect the physical realm immediately. Repentance of a human heart is followed by immediate forgiveness from God's throne. It is a spiritual law. Repentance removes condemnation and positions the contrite person back on the narrow road for eternity with Jesus.

King David knew the power of repentance and practiced it. He recorded his experience in Psalm 51:17, when the prophet Nathan came to him after King David had committed adultery with Bathsheba.

> My sacrifice, O God, is a broken spirit; a broken and contrite heart you, God, will not despise. (Psalms 51:17)

We, the believers in Christ, are not in a different position from the Israelites or King David on the issue of being prone to the enslaving power of sin. Jews and Gentiles alike are all under the power of sin (Romans 3:9), says the Apostle Paul. This power was deadly for the Israelites, and it is deadly for us as well. The Lord cried then, calling His people to turn back to Him. The Lord continues to cry after us even today, saying,

> Be earnest, and repent! Here I am! I stand at the door and knock. If anyone hears my voice and opens the door, I will come in and eat with him, and he with me. (Revelation 3:19b-20)

Note who Lord Jesus calls to repent, not the lost out in the world, but those who already have been redeemed! Why would the Lord call the already saved? For the same reason that He called the Israelites to turn from their evil ways. The Lord God does not want any of His own to die on account of sin (Ezekiel 33:11). Repentance has the power to cancel a death sentence of sin and turn it into a blessing of life. Take Jesus' call for repentance seriously, be earnest, and repent (Revelation 3:19)!

Confession and Repentance—The Key to Healing

Prayer for healing starts with confession and repentance. God hears a wholehearted confession and forgives. This is a spiritual Law. You must understand that when you confess and repent wholeheartedly, you are indeed forgiven. Your mouth has spoken words representing thoughts and attitudes deep within your heart. Let no doubts trouble your mind and torment your soul. Let your mind and heart come to complete agreement with this fact: The moment you pray for forgiveness, God forgives you. The moment you confess and repent, God wipes it out. His forgiveness is immediate. Everything else is a lie from the pit of hell.

Jesus did not take a month, a week, a day, or even an hour to grant you forgiveness when you first repented and were saved. The very moment when you confess with your mouth, "Jesus is Lord," and believe in your heart that God raised him from the dead, you are saved (Romans 10:9). So it is with confessing our sins after we have entered the Kingdom of God.

> If we confess our sins, he is faithful and just and will forgive us
>
> our sins and purify us from all unrighteousness. (1 John 1:9)

The enemy's biggest target is the believer walking on the narrow road toward eternity with Jesus. The Devil is like a thief in the night (John 10:10), like a prowling lion looking for someone to devour (1 Peter 5:8). Sin weakens the armor of God, giving the Devil an "open door" access to harm the believer (Ephesians 4:26-27). Confession and repentance from sin close that door immediately, preventing any attack from being successful.

Question: When was the last time you confessed and repented?

_____

_____

_____

_____

_____

_____

Two Goats and The Cross

The Old Testament sacrificial system is a shadow of the sacrifice of Christ (Hebrews 10:1). The daily Temple practices were quite elaborate, but on the Day of Atonement, Aaron had to perform an extra duty: From the Israelite community, he was to take two identical, male goats, and casting lots determined which one would be a sin offering to the Lord and which would be the scapegoat, known as Azazel (Leviticus 16:7-22). For non-holiday Temple practices, the blood of the sacrificial animal, presented before the Lord, constituted a sin offering for the forgiveness of the sins of Israel. On the Day of Atonement, that alone was not sufficient. The sins had to be separated from the people. The second goat, Azazel—the scapegoat—served the purpose. The high priest was to put both his hands on the head of the goat and evoke all the sins of Israel, transferring them to the Azazel goat. The goat is then taken to the desert to die, thus separating the sin from the people forever. This is an act of removing defilement among the people of Israel, and only with the banishment of the goat, the atonement is considered final. The psalmist recorded this spiritual mystery.

> As far as the east is from the west, so far has he removed our
> transgressions from us. (Psalms 103:12)

In chapter ten, the author of Hebrews discusses these practices at length, weighing them against the ultimate sacrifice of Jesus.

> Those sacrifices are an annual reminder of sins because it is
> impossible for the blood of bulls and goats to take away the
> sins. ... Day after day, every priest stands and performs his
> religious duties; again and again he offers the same sacrifices,
> which can never take away sins. (Hebrews 10:3,11)

He further contrasts the sacrifice of Jesus, who, through His death on the cross, made perfect forever those who are being made holy (Hebrews 10:14). The sacrifice of Jesus on the cross satisfied the purpose of the two goats on the Day of Atonement. The cross of Jesus serves the double functions of the two goats:

1) Atonement for sins through the blood of Jesus spilled on the cross;
   God presented him as a sacrifice of atonement through faith in
   his blood. (Romans 3:25)

In him, we have redemption through his blood, the forgiveness of sins, according to the riches of God's grace. (Ephesians 1:7)

To him who loves us and has freed us from our sins by his blood. (Revelation 1:5b)

Now we can enter, without fear, the Most holy Place by the blood of Jesus. (Hebrews 10:19)

2) Separation from sins through nailing them on the cross and declaring them dead. Similarly, like the Azazel goat, all the sins of the world were placed on Jesus as He suffered on the cross.

The next day, he saw Jesus coming toward him and said, "Behold, the Lamb of God, who takes away the sin of the world!" (John 1:29)

He forgave us all our sins, having canceled the written code, with its regulations, that was against us that stood opposed to us; he took it away, nailing it to the cross. (Colossians 2:14)

So Christ was sacrificed once to take away the sins of many people, and he will appear a second time, not to bear sin but to bring salvation to those waiting for him. (Hebrews 9:28)

The cross of Jesus is the substitute for the Azazel goat. God has laid on Jesus the iniquity of us all (Isaiah 53:6). On the cross, Jesus bore all the sins of the world, every sin of every sinner ever committed.

God made him to be sin who had no sin, to be sin for us, so that in him we might become the righteousness of God. (2 Corinthians 5:21)

Forgiveness starts with confession and ends with repentance. Healing requires total separation from sins.

He himself bore our sins in his body on the tree, that we might die to sin and live to righteousness; by his wounds you have been healed. (1 Peter 2:24)

There is no other way to separate from our sins but the way of the cross of Jesus. The contemporaries of Jesus could not understand when He said,

> I am the way and the truth and the life. No one comes to the
> Father except through me. (John 14:6)

Today, we are privileged to know the deep things of God. It will be ignorance if we do not apply 1) the blood for forgiveness and cleansing, and 2) the cross for the removal of sin and sanctification. The healing from traumatic events requires the practice of both. This is a spiritual transaction. Unlike the ancient Israelites, we don't need the continuous spilling of the blood of sacrificial animals. The claim of the cleansing power of the blood of Jesus spilled on the cross evokes its purifying power. Similarly, we nail our sins on the cross and claim the power of the cross to separate us from our inequity for eternity (see detailed description and prayers in session six). Once claimed, the matter is done on earth as it is in heaven.

The Traps of Resentment, Bitterness, Hatred, and Anger

You, suffering from emotional pain, may say, "Why must I repent? I haven't done anything wrong, but wrong has been done to me. I am a victim. I am in pain. I need healing. What does repentance have to do with my pain? I should be getting apologies, not being asked to apologize!" Yes, you have the right to feel the way you do: Bitter and angry towards the perpetrator and resentful towards your offender. This is the most "natural" response to any assault. The secular world validates these feelings. You, most likely, have held this position and consequently have exercised your right to be bitter and angry for how many long years _____? Now, this is what the Lord Himself tells you,

> I take no pleasure in the death of anyone, declares the
> Sovereign LORD. Repent and live! (Ezekiel 18:32)

A response of fury and indignation is warranted here: How could victims heap death on their souls? How could victims of injustice share the same punishment as the offenders? Let's consider turning to the Scripture for answers. What have you gained from being angry, bitter, and resentful? The Apostle Paul says,

> Do not be deceived: God cannot be mocked. A man reaps what he sows. The one who sows to please his sinful nature, from that nature will reap destruction; the one who sows to please the Spirit, from the Spirit will reap eternal life. (Galatians 6:7-8)

What have you been reaping for the last (how many) ____ long years? Bitterness? Resentment? Anger? Do you realize that what you have sown are the seeds of these same attitudes deep in your heart? Do you know that engaging in these practices has allowed them to grow roots deep inside your soul? They have become part of your character. Are you now happy with the harvest? No, sowing a "handful" of bitterness brought you "bushels" of tears and desperation, figuratively speaking. Your pain is further exacerbated; it has turned into intolerable misery. Like the Israelites, you groan, "I am wasting away." And like them, you are more likely to refuse to recognize the root problem of your condition, which is the lack of repentance from the sin of bitterness, anger, animosity, hate, and resentment. Sowing and reaping is a spiritual law. The secular world refers to it as karma.

The Bible gives us a simple spiritual rule: If a bad fruit is present in the believer's life, undead flesh is "feeding" on unrepentant sin. Bitterness, resentment, animosity, and anger are bad fruits in the life of a believer. They are red flags, warning of a "breached security" in the armor of God. How long is one able to resist the incessant attacks of the enemy before the Devil takes a foothold (Ephesians 4:27-29) in the heart and begins his evil work of kill, steal, and destroy (John 10:10)? The best protection strategy of the believer is to be armed with the knowledge of how to thwart these attacks. Again, it is straightforward: Repentance from bitterness, resentment, and anger closes all access doors, thus denying the enemy legal permission to enter and stay. The warning to us is stern:

See to it that no one falls short of the grace of God and that no bitter root grows up to cause trouble and defile many. (Hebrews 12:15)

Don't sow bitterness, resentment, and anger so you won't reap their bitter fruit. Don't be involved in these sinful practices of the flesh, and you will see how their wickedness will flee you. Instead, do what Jesus said those who abide in Him are to do:

Love your enemies, and pray for those who persecute you, that you may be sons of your Father in heaven. (Matthew 5:44)

Instead of resentment and bitterness, the Apostle Paul advises us to put into practice an opposite attitude.

Let us not become weary in doing good, for at the proper time, we will reap a harvest if we do not give up. Therefore, as we have opportunity, let us do good to all people, especially to those who belong to the family of believers. (Galatians 6:9-10)

Regarding your perpetrator, consider the biblical advice to show goodness towards the offender,

You will heap burning coals on their heads, and the LORD will reward you. (Proverbs 25:22)

Your healing is not in vengeful thoughts and bitter emotions. The key to beginning the process of healing is repentance from them! No one can escape from prison unless the fortified walls have been weakened from inside.

As no one is discharged in time of war, so wickedness will not release those who practice it. (Ecclesiastes 8:8b)

Wickedness will flee if one repents, renounces, and hauls it to the cross, declaring it dead. Bitterness, resentment, hatred, and anger are the wickedness you must release through repentance and death on the cross. They don't exist in the Kingdom of God; they should not be part of a believer's life either. The prison walls you are held behind are the walls built by your own sin, and the war you are engaged in is a war of life and death. How you come out of this war depends on how you deal with sin. Sin does not release those who practice it, only those who renounce it and repent from it. "Repent, for the kingdom of heaven is near," were the first words John the Baptist preached (Matthew 3:2). "Repent, for the kingdom of heaven is near," were also the first words Jesus preached at the beginning of His ministry (Matthew 4:17). Jesus sent out the twelve disciples with the instruction to preach repentance and heal the sick (Mark 6:12,13). And when the cities that witnessed Jesus' miracles remained unrepentant, He denounced them (Matthew 11:20).

The key to entering the Kingdom of God is repentance. The key to remaining in the Kingdom of God is the practice of daily repentance.

Something happens in the heavenly realm when we approach God with a broken spirit. We are considered blessed, and we are allowed to enter the Kingdom of God (Matthew 5:3). God passes judgment if we say, "I haven't sinned" (Jeremiah 2:35). But, if we confess our sins, he is faithful and just and will forgive us our sins and purify us from all unrighteousness (1 John 1:9). This is what the Sovereign Lord, the Holy One of Israel, says,

> In repentance and rest is your salvation, in quietness and trust
> is your strength. (Isaiah 30:15)

King David was a man after God's own heart. His wholehearted repentance from sin brought him this position despite his many faults. King David articulated his own experience with sin and repentance:

> Blessed is he whose transgressions are forgiven, whose sins
> are covered. Blessed is the man whose sin the LORD does not
> count against him and in whose spirit is no deceit. When I
> kept silent, my bones wasted away through my groaning all
> day long. For day and night your hand was heavy upon me; my
> strength was sapped as in the heat of summer. Then I
> acknowledged my sin to you and did not cover up my iniquity.
> I said, "I will confess my transgressions to the LORD" – and

you forgave the guilt of my sin. Therefore, let everyone who is godly pray to You while You may be found. (Psalms 32:1-6)

The Lord can be found, and His Word can indeed still the raging waters of life. He calls us to enter into His presence, where the rising storm is silenced before it becomes a threat and where the provisions for the journey on the narrow road are never depleted. The Lord God is never weary of crying out after His children.

Come, all you who are thirsty, come to the waters; and you who have no money, come, buy and eat! Come, buy wine and milk without money and without cost. Why spend money on what is not bread, and your labor on what does not satisfy? Listen, listen to me, and eat what is good, and your soul will delight in the richest of fare. Give ear and come to me; hear me, that your soul may live. (Isaiah 55:1-3)

Angry With God

Do all people who have experienced traumatic events exhibit anger toward God? Becoming angry with God is a spontaneous reaction of Christians and non-Christians alike. The first group trusted in God's sovereign protection, and the incident of trauma left them with feelings of betrayal and uncertainty, with questions echoing night and day, "Why? Where were you, God?" There is an irony in the possibility that the closer the relationship with God is before the traumatic event, the stronger the anger with God becomes afterward. The betrayal of a trustworthy friend (God) is harrowing and becomes a trauma of its own. This attitude, however, becomes an impediment to spiritual growth.

For the second group, the lack of God's involvement only confirms the belief that "If God is good, how could He allow such things to happen? Does He care? Does He even exist?" While, in this situation, the nonbeliever displays the attitude of a fool (Romans 1:18-23), the believer has no excuse to measure up to the same folly. And yet, in the Church, we see more often a full display of Cain's predicament rather than Job's predicament.

The Scripture doesn't specify why God looked favorably at Abel's offering but not at Cain's (Genesis 1:1). Some clues bring understanding. The story tells us that,

> So Cain was very angry, and his face was downcast. Then the
> LORD said to Cain, "Why are you angry? Why is your face
> downcast?" (Genesis 4:5b-6a)

The very next comment God made to Cain, "If you do what is right, will you not be accepted?" (Genesis 4:6), leads to the understanding that apparently, Cain did not "walk in integrity of heart and in uprightness" (1 Kings 9:4-5) and he did not do what was "right in the eyes of the Lord" (1 Kings 15:15). God has repeatedly rejected the offerings, the prayers and the fasts of worshipers in whom such conditions of heart and mind were present (Isaiah 1:11-15, Isaiah 58:3-5; Jeremiah 6:20; Amos 5:21–23). Instead, God desires mercy, not sacrifice, and acknowledgment of God rather than burnt offerings (Hosea 6:6).

Cain's anger with God arose out of jealousy. Deep in his heart, the seed of sin sprouted bitterness. Anger and rage followed, quickly escalating into premeditated murder (Genesis 4:8). Because Cain did not do what was right in the sight of God, he became vulnerable to the influence of the evil forces in the spiritual realm. He gave the enemy a "foothold" (Ephesians 4:27-29) to steal, kill, and destroy (John 10:10). He became a murderer long before he killed his brother Abel because the Scripture defines the one who hates his brother as a murderer (1 John 3:15-17; Matthew 5:21-22). Even though the Law of Moses was given to humanity long after the murder of Abel, the spiritual laws that govern God's creation had contained these precepts since the beginning of time. Cain's actions were judged against God's eternal spiritual laws and were found sinful.

Cain failed to master the constant attacks of the powers of darkness that drove him to act out treacherously. The Scripture describes those attacks as sin, crouching at his door and desiring to have him (Genesis 4:7). Cain did not master the sin; he became enslaved by the sin; he became a symbol of sin.

After committing the murder, Cain had no regrets. He did not confess, nor did he repent from his actions. His rebellion brought him a curse (Genesis 4:11). Cain followed in the footsteps of his father, Adam, and his mother, Eve, who failed to acknowledge their wrongdoing, tried to cover their offense, and never regretted their actions (Genesis 3:8-13). In both cases, rebellious attitudes of the heart and a bold denial of actions are present, resulting in an identical outcome of being cast out of God's presence. This is Cain's predicament.

Compared to Cain, Job had more "justifiable" reasons to be angry with God. Cain had no adverse events (trauma) in his life, while Job's trauma was enormous, losing everything dear to him—all of his children, wealth, health, and dignity. And yet, we are seeing two completely different manifestations of anger with God that led to two opposite eternal outcomes.

Behind the scenes, in Job's story, we are given insights into how the enemy operates in the spiritual realm, enticing, tormenting, and plotting the ultimate annihilation of the soul. We also see that even in its ugly rage, the enemy can only do what God allows him to do (Job 1:12; 2:6). The end goal of Satan is to cause Job to curse God to his face (Job 2:5), and thus be destined to hell rather than eternity with God. Job didn't sin against God. He endured the days of trouble.

Job's story gives the believer a blueprint for processing and handling anger with God. Anger is an emotion imparted to us since the beginning of time. God exhibits anger, and yet God is holy. Since we are created in His image, we can also be angry and not sin. Apostle Paul acknowledged this dichotomy, warning us not to sin in our anger (Ephesians 4:26). How do we practically comply with this instruction?

Question: What fuels my anger? What are the situations, individuals, or things that make me angry?

_____

_____

_____

Now, compare your response to what fuels God's anger and discuss how they measure up compared to your triggers. God's wrath rages at injustice (Proverbs 17:15), dishonesty (Proverbs 11:1), wickedness (Romans 1:18), and disobedience (1 Kings 11:9-10). Jesus burst with anger at the moneychangers, driving them out of the temple of God. Yet, He didn't sin.

> "My house will be called a house of prayer," but you are making it a den of robbers. (Matthew 21:13b)

Every thought, attitude of heart, and action contrary to God's will on earth and heaven (Matthew 6:10) is detestable to Him. His anger is fueled by unjust practices (Amos 5:24), a divine indignation. Just like God, we are instructed to hate what is evil and cling to what is good (Romans 12:9). This understanding produces in us the same divine indignation in which there is no sin. Everything else is from the enemy.

Many believers whose lives are affected by traumatic events may disassociate with Job's story, thinking, I am not innocent like Job; I deserve God's discipline, and I must accept His punishment. Yes, it might be the case in which you, just like Cain, through actions or attitudes of heart, have opened a door, giving a foothold to the enemy to wreak havoc on your life. But this is where Cain's predicament ends. Your story doesn't have to end here. If you find yourself in Cain's position of sinning against God, do not despair; God has given us a way to right the wrong, remove the stains, and be victorious in overcoming the Devil's schemes. It is the ancient way of humbling oneself before the Almighty God, confessing sin, and seeking His forgiveness.

> If my people, who are called by my name, will humble themselves and pray and seek my face and turn from their

wicked ways, then I will hear from heaven, and I will forgive

their sin and will heal their land. (2 Chronicles 7:14)

Job followed the above pattern in dealing with grief and bitterness in response to the traumatic events in his life. This pattern is beneficial for believers affected by traumatic events who harbor anger toward God.

1. Have an enduring faith in God. In times of calamity, Job held strong onto his faith. He knew God's just character. He had a close relationship with Him.

I know that my Redeemer lives and that in the end, he will

stand on the earth. And after my skin has been destroyed, yet

in my flesh I will see God; I myself will see him with my own

eyes—I, and not another. How my heart yearns within me!

(Job 19:25-27)

Job's story is like Abraham's—a story of testing the faith. Tragedies struck Job; Abraham was told to sacrifice his only son. Job could not understand why God would allow such an enormous suffering to fall upon him, but nevertheless, he trusted the Lord.

Though he slay me, yet will I hope in him. (Job 13:15)

I know I will be vindicated. (Job 13:18)

Likewise, Abraham could not understand why God would demand such a cruel action from him, but he trusted the Lord.

Abraham answered, "God himself will provide the lamb for the burnt offering, my son." (Genesis 22:8)

These two men exemplify the strength of faith in times of crisis. They both passed the test, which was credited to them as righteousness (Genesis 15:6; Job 42:7b).

2. Be honest with God. Job continuously defended his innocence. With long orations, his friends tried to convince him otherwise, urging him to acknowledge his sins and accept God's just punishment. Even his wife said to him, "Are you still maintaining your integrity? Curse God and die!" (Job 2:9)

Job couldn't completely understand why all these evil things were happening to him. In the anguish of his heart, Job cried out to God, asking for an audience with Him to argue his case of innocence.

> But I desire to speak to the Almighty and to argue my case
> with God. (Job 13:3)

God listened to Job's arguments and vindicated his case. Amid the crisis and despite all the negativism around him, Job remained blameless and upright (Job 2:3). In his dealings with God, Job displayed an array of emotions, including anger (Job 18:4), and yet,

> In all this, Job did not sin by charging God with wrongdoing.
> (Job 1:22)

Job's story encourages us to approach God and talk to Him in the anguish of our own suffering. Just like Job, God will speak to us out of the storm (Job 38:1). On this side of eternity, we might never get satisfactory answers to our questions. But, this is where we display the strength and integrity of faith to

> Trust in the LORD with all your heart and lean not on your
> own understanding; in all your ways submit to him, and he
> will make your paths straight. (Proverbs 3:5-6)

3. Be humbled before God. God spoke with Job and made him utterly aware of how absolutely awesome He is. Job understood God's place and his own standing in the divinely created order, and Job grew in appreciation. He recognized the pitiful position he found himself in, acknowledging,

> My ears had heard of you, but now my eyes have seen you.
> Therefore, I despise myself and repent in dust and ashes. (Job
> 42:5-6)

Job repented and was restored. This is Job's predicament. We should all follow suit and make it our predicament. Knowingly or unknowingly, we are also prone to sin against God, especially in the misery of our pain and suffering. It is difficult to make eye contact with someone we deeply judge in our hearts because of the overwhelming presence of animosity, bitterness, and anger. How much more difficult is it when we harbor these toward God? Like Job, we must acknowledge, and like the Prophet Isaiah, we must admit:

> Yet you, LORD, are our Father. We are the clay, you are the potter; we are all the work of your hand. (Isaiah 64:8)

Question: Were you able to attend services, pray, or worship the Lord at the time of your trauma? Compare your ability to worship God right now.

The Story of Lea

For a long time, the news could not penetrate Lea's head. It hung outside her consciousness, denying acknowledgment. The heart, however, buckled under these horrible words, penetrating deep, piercing with pain: "Your son just died." Her face turned pale; drained of any strength, her body crumpled motionless to the ground.

Tears flowed day and night as waves of pain were folding her in spasmodic convulsions, sapping the last bits of energy. But, even then, sleep evaded her. Rest was far from her. The eerie silence of many sleepless nights threw Lea's mind reeling at high velocity. "Why, God?" she cried silently, only to be met with equal silence.

Lea knew she was losing her peace. Prayers, studies and devotionals were far from the capability of her mind to engage in them. She could not get herself to face God in prayer. Attending worship on Sunday terrified her. And then, a familiar pattern emerged: A Bible verse emerged in her mind, delivering a message, illuminating an understanding.

> The righteous perish, and no one ponders in his heart; the devout men are taken away, and no one understands that the righteous are taken away to be spared from evil. (Isaiah 57:1)

Lea knew that God had spoken. The message, though informative, didn't bring her the desired relief but piled more unanswered questions. She felt robbed of the joy of not having her boy in this world. All the plans and hopes built together had suddenly vanished. A deep void lodged within her heart, stealing away the small joys of life. Prayer time was tough. She would call God's name and remain in His presence, weeping silently. A reverent fear rose steadily within her—a fear of being angry with God. Throughout the years, God has delivered answers to Lea's countless prayers, performing signs and miracles of healing, building her faith steadily into a giant mountain. His investments in her life were paying off now. Lea embraced Job's attitude of suffering.

> The LORD gave, and the LORD has taken away; may the name
> of the LORD be praised. (Job 1:21)

Months have passed with no relief from the pain. One Sunday, after service, her heart was weighty with sorrow. She just wanted to be away, left alone for some time, to spare her family from watching her in this miserable condition. The choice was not difficult to make. Her family was in the process of building their dream home just a few miles away. The still unfinished back porch was her preferred place for seclusion in prayer. As Lea headed towards the ranch, tears began rolling down her sad face. A deep longing in her heart rose, a strong desire to be with her mother at that very moment, a yearning to fall in her arms and cry her heart out on her shoulder. But her mother was thousands of miles away; she knew her desire was unattainable.

As she turned onto the private dirt road, she noticed another car heading in the same direction right before her. The people were either lost or were going to the ranch; the alternatives were apparent, Lea thought. Sure enough, the vehicle began climbing the small hill, advancing towards the building site. Both cars came to a stop side-by-side. A couple rolled down the window and began apologizing, explaining that they knew the building contractor who had spoken highly of the design and the house's location and had encouraged them to visit the site. They were in the neighborhood, they said, visiting a relative and decided to swing by to see the beauty for themselves.

Lea's plans for seclusion had to wait. She extended hospitality to the couple and took them on a tour as they marveled at the unique features she showed them. The tour ended at the back porch. The flood of sorrow was now an unrelentless pounding on her soul. Lea broke down in tears, unable to hold the crushing weight, as she revealed her heavy heart to the two strangers. Without saying a word, the woman stepped forward and gently embraced Lea. For a long moment, Lea gave in to her sorrows and wept quietly on the woman's shoulder. "It is my shoulder. It is my comfort for you, Lea," the Lord whispered.

Later that night, Lea pondered in awe about God's extraordinary providence. That afternoon, God arranged all events perfectly, bringing people and resources in perfect order and timing to deliver the desired comfort and message: "I love you, Lea." It was just a longing, not even a voiced prayer, and yet, God knew the need and immediately delivered the relief, proving once again the truthfulness of the Scripture.

> In the same way, the Spirit helps us in our weakness. We do not know what we ought to pray for, but the Spirit himself intercedes for us with groans that words cannot express. And he who searches our hearts knows the mind of the Spirit, because the Spirit intercedes for the saints in accordance with God's will. (Romans 8:26-27)

To this day, Lea's sorrow continues to be a part of her life. The debilitating sting of pain, however, was gone. The arms of the woman were a conduit of God's healing power for Lea. In all her sorrowful experiences, Lea did not sin against God. The fear of offending Him by questioning her fate was the wisdom from above she acquired along the many years of an intimate relationship with Jesus. God responded with a favor, bestowing a blessing on her and her family. Lea had another son, a daily reminder of her firstborn, now in heaven for eternity with the Lord.

Four Basic Spiritual Laws

Any form of abuse is a double murder. First, its judgment stands against the offender who committed the wrongdoing, convicting them of sin. At the same time, it provokes a sinful reaction from the victim who suffered the offense. The reaction is a self-defense mechanism against the abuser with the end goal of survival. Hatred and anger towards the perpetrator are the most natural responses of a victim. When the abuse persists over a longer period, these reactions become fixed psychological constructs set in the mind of the individual. Hatred and anger become part of the individual's character. At this point, these are not only mere psychological constructs but curses associated with violating four basic spiritual laws.

Spiritual Law 1: Honor your father and your mother, as the Lord your God has commanded you. So that you may live long and that it may go well with you in the land the Lord your God is giving you. (Deuteronomy 5:16)

Spiritual Law 2: Do not be deceived; God is not mocked; for whatever a man sows, this he will also reap. (Galatians 6:7)

Spiritual Law 3: Do not judge, or you too will be judged. For in the same way you judge others, you will be judged, and with the measure you use, it will be measured to you. (Matthew 7:1-2)

Spiritual Law 4: For if you forgive other people when they sin against you, your heavenly Father will also forgive you. (Matthew 6:14; Luke 6:37)

With time, resentment, bitterness, hatred, and anger become part of a person's personality. They become engraved psychological constructs through which we engage the world around us. They are practices of the old nature, of the flesh. How do we liberate ourselves from the enslaving power of the flesh that has now become part of our character? The Church sacrament of penitence is a divine tool for healing:

1) Repent and renounce the identified practices of the flesh.

2) Extend forgiveness towards those who caused you pain

3) Repent from your reactions to the offense

4) Crucify the practices of the flesh; call to death on the cross the root of anger, resentment, and bitterness.

5) Take authority in Christ to break the power of the psychological construct over your mind and heart, knowing that "whatever you bind on earth will be bound in heaven, and whatever you loose on earth will be loosed in heaven." (Matthew 16:19; 18:18)

6) Wash in the blood of Jesus for purification of mind and body, soul and spirit. What has been touched by evil and become defiled must be washed pure by the blood of Jesus spilled on the cross.

7) Fill up with the Holy Spirit

8) Call to life a new way of responding, consistent with the Kingdom of God.

The steps above cancel the curses associated with these laws; they no longer have power over the life of a believer. Once the root problem is identified, it has to be renounced, and forgiveness needs to be extended to the individual(s) who caused this seed to be sown and take root in the heart.

Prayer for breaking psychological constructs

Jesus, I recognize the destructive power of bitterness, resentment, anger, and hatred over my life. Thank you for granting me an understanding of the captivity I have been subjected to. I now choose to reject these practices of the flesh. Forgive me, Jesus. I take to the cross these practices of the flesh, and I crucify them, condemning them to death. I declare them separated from me for eternity. I apply your blood, Jesus, spilled on the cross to cleanse me from the defiling presence of these sinful practices. Bring into my life new ways of responding to people who hurt me. Jesus, I was not aware that by judging my parents, I have dishonored them. Forgive my ignorance, Lord. I now wholeheartedly forgive my parents for _____. I pray that You now restore to me the blessings of life. I pray against the stronghold of _____ in my life, and I break free from its dominion. I pray in the name of my Lord, God, and Savior, Jesus Christ. Amen!

EHAD with GOD

REFLECTION—Week Five

Reflection 1: Give Him 5—a daily practice of God's presence (see description on pages 41 and 63 under "Deep calls to deep" section)

Reflection 2: Daily confession and repentance in prayer to Christ—our high priest; crucify the flesh, wash with the blood, fill with the Holy Spirit (page 13)

Reflection 3: How do I measure against the four basic spiritual laws?

Reflection 4: The Power of the Spoken Word—The Story of Peter

Question: How do I measure against the four basic spiritual laws?

Honor your father and your mother

_____

_____

_____

_____

Whatever a man sows, this he will also reap

_____

_____

_____

_____

Do not judge, or you too will be judged

_____

_____

_____

_____

Forgive others so that your heavenly Father will also forgive you

_____

_____

_____

_____

Forgiveness—The Story of Peter

Peter sought counseling for his anger outbursts. Uncontrollable and unpredictable episodes of rage damaged every area of his life. Peter was a believer in Jesus Christ. His sins were forgiven, and he strived for goodness but could not achieve it. On Sundays, he felt sorrowfully repentant and readily made new promises to God for radical changes. Despite Sunday's assertion, Mondays proved to be another failure for Peter to conform to a truthful life in Christ. As a result, Peter grew angrier with himself and the world around him. It was out of this deepening frustration that Peter finally took the advice of a church elder and considered getting help.

Prayer counseling identified the root of bitterness and anger. Peter harbored resentment towards his parents, which was seeded in his early childhood. Peter was born with a physical impairment, which his parents considered embarrassing and damaging to their social image. As a young child, Peter grew up isolated, kept behind locked doors and shut down windows. He was unjustifiably deprived of childhood's simple joys. During his school years, Peter's seclusion continued to grow, fed by his schoolmates' cruelty and some of his teachers' insensitivities towards his handicap. Deep in his heart, Peter judged his parents for causing him undeserved pain, and he hated his schoolmates and teachers, who further aggravated his suffering.

Peter did not shrivel in pain but fought against his misery by imploring a compensatory mechanism, which counteracted the absence of love, attention, and recognition in his life. Peter strove for and achieved academic excellence. From an early school age, he realized he had a brilliant mind. His intelligence became the source of attention and recognition he desperately desired. Peter began to enjoy his mind's power over people and found it easy to manipulate them for his own benefit. He became arrogant. His arrogance, though, did not propel him through his university studies; he was not so easily distinguished among many other equally brilliant young men and women. When he could not gain people's recognition through hard academic work, Peter's rage and arrogance turned against them. His friendships were minefields of broken promises and failed relationships. He could not retain employment, and all dealings associated with it were eroded.

While on the surface, he was arrogant, deep inside, Peter felt lonely and hurt. He longed for closeness, but his machinations drove prospective companions away. This further enraged Peter and hard-pressed him towards alcohol use for consolation. It was after a night of overindulgence that Peter wrecked his pickup truck and was arrested for driving under the influence of alcohol.

Let's look at Peter's story while applying the four basic spiritual laws. Peter dishonored his mother and father by judging them. According to the law, life will not go well for Peter in the area in which he dishonored his parents. He judged them for being cruel to him. In his adult life, Peter's arrogance, bordered with cruelty, made him openly hostile towards his fellow students and coworkers. His relationship with his parents was scarred with bitterness and resentment. The relationships with his peers also bore the same hallmark.

Peter responded to his parents' mistreatment with bitterness. It took deep root in his heart and sprang the seed of anger and arrogance. Peter's reaction to his parents' sin was, likewise, sinful. The law is impersonal, and its just retributions reach Peter even though he was an innocent victim of circumstance. It was not the emotional pain caused by his parents that made him sin; it was his embittered reaction towards them that accused him of wrongdoing. The sin of bitterness enslaved Peter.

To break from the enslaving power of sin, Peter had to satisfy the just retribution of the law by confessing his wrongful behavior and forgiving those who sinned against him. Peter had to forgive his parents to receive healing from anger and resentment. Repentance from the sin of bitterness and forgiveness towards those who sinned against him freed Peter from the emotional pain he suffered. By extending forgiveness to his offenders, Peter was on the road to healing from his miserable condition of heart; his misery soon turned to serene peace.

I Choose to Forgive: Life of Hate and Misery vs. Life of Freedom

Question: What is your strategy to win this battle? Do you find similarities between Peter's story and your story? Write your own prayer for liberation from unforgiveness.

_____
_____
_____
_____
_____
_____
_____
_____
_____
_____
_____
_____
_____
_____
_____
_____
_____
_____
_____
_____
_____
_____
_____
_____
_____
_____
_____
_____
_____
_____
_____

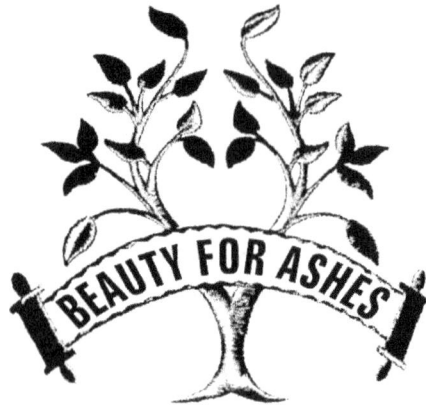

SESSION SIX

KEEP THE SABBATH HOLY

Every day, Jesus was at the Temple, under the Solomon colonnade, teaching the people who gathered around him (John 10:23). He spoke of many spiritual things, and very few understood him. But when he said, "I will give you rest," they knew what He was talking about; every Jewish person knew the spiritual meaning of his appeal.

> "Come to me, all you who are weary and burdened, and I will give you rest. Take my yoke upon you and learn from me, for I am gentle and humble in heart, and you will find rest for your souls. For my yoke is easy and my burden is light." (Matthew 11:28-30)

For today's culture, Jesus' call for "rest" is understood as physical rest from labor, resting on the couch, watching a favorite show, or enjoying favorite activities, such as fishing or gardening, for example. For the Israelites of Jesus' time, "rest" meant the Sabbath Day rest. There are two Hebrew words for "rest" —"sabbath" (שבת) and "menuha" (מנוחה). They both mean physical rest with the emphasis on spiritual rest for the soul (Matthew 11:30). The meaning is derived from the creation story in Genesis 2:3, where God, after creating everything in six days, rested (shabbat) from His labor on the seventh day.

> By the seventh day God had finished the work he had been doing; so on the seventh day he **rested** [שבת, sabbath] from all his work. Then God blessed the seventh day and made it holy, because in it he **rested** [שבת, sabbath] from all the work of creating that he had done. (Genesis 2:3)

Why would God rest? Was he tired from his labor? The Scripture tells us otherwise.

> The LORD is the everlasting God, the creator of the ends of the earth. He will not grow tired or weary. (Isaiah 40:28)
> Indeed, he who watches over Israel will neither slumber nor sleep. (Psalms 121:4)

So, it is clear that Genesis 2:3 doesn't refer to a rest from physical exhaustion. What kind of rest is it then?

> This is what the LORD says: "Heaven is my throne, and the earth is my footstool. Where is the house you will build for me? Where will my resting place [menuhati] be? (Isaiah 66:1)

Is Isaiah referring to the Temple in Jerusalem as a resting place for God? Or, is there a deeper meaning of God's rest?

One Sabbath, Jesus was walking through the fields with his disciples, and they, being hungry, began to pick some heads of grain and eat them. The Pharisees judged this act as unlawful on the Sabbath day. In their defense, Jesus responded that the Sabbath was made for man, not man for the Sabbath (Mark 2:27; Luke 6:5). The seventh day is called "the Sabbath of the LORD" (Exodus 20:8-10). The phrase "of the LORD" connotes possession. It is the

Lord's day! Yet, God didn't bless and hallow the Sabbath for himself, but for humankind. What is, then, God's rest? What constitutes God's rest/Sabbath? What is Jesus implying when He said, "I will give you rest"? To answer these questions, we must go back to the Genesis story (Genesis 2:3).

Entropy Mode

At the Fall of Adam and Eve, the whole creation became corrupted, humans and nature alike began steadily going into an entropy mode—from degradation and disintegration to total annihilation. Apostle Paul writes,

> For this world in its present form is passing away.

(1 Corinthians 7:31b)

The Sabbath Day, however, is not part of God's natural creation. The Sabbath Day is a time period, a time capsule, an event, or a concept that is not affected by the decay of the physical realm. The Sabbath Day cannot be corrupted. Time stands outside the natural laws. God blessed the "time" of the Sabbath and made it holy. Thus, the holiness of the Sabbath day has remained even after the Fall of humankind and nature; the holiness of the Sabbath endures to this day. The Sabbath Day is a blessed and holy time sanctuary of God's presence. To this day, God continues to rest (sabbath) on the seventh day; God is present on the seventh day. It is a spiritual law established at the time of creation. When we adhere to the call to enter His rest, we are invited to enter the sacred time sanctuary of God and meet with Him on the Sabbath Day. This is His indestructible temple of time, which neither the Babylonians nor the Romans, nor the Atheism of the Communists can destroy.

The Holiness of the Shabbat

Why did God single out a special day to be holy, since everything in the Garden of Eden was holy? God created the world in perfect holiness; everything in the Garden of Eden was holy, untouched by sin. God walked in the cool of the day in the garden with Adam and Eve, in face-to-face fellowship. There was no temple in the Garden of Eden. The whole creation was God's temple. God was its temple. The Fall changed the course of human history. God, who is holy, remained holy while the human race became defiled. The Scripture tells us that "without holiness no one will see God" (Hebrews 12:14). The face-to-face fellowship no longer was sustained. No longer could one see God and remain alive (Exodus 33:20).

Adam was not commanded to keep the Sabbath. Adam was created holy, compatible with the holiness of the Sabbath. Since he was not defiled, he was in God's holy presence perpetually, not only on the seventh day. Only after the Fall, and only after God chose the Hebrew nation out of all the families on earth, did He reintroduce Himself through the holiness of the Sabbath for holy communion with mankind.

The Sabbath Day is God's divine providence for humanity to encounter His holiness under the corrupt circumstances after the Fall. Before creating the world, God foresaw the Fall. He also foresaw Jesus with His mission for the redemption of humanity (Ephesians 1:4), and He foresaw all individuals who would say "yes" to Him and be saved (1 Peter 1:20). God knew we would fail before He spoke the world into being. The Sabbath Day is God's divine providence for humanity to have access to God's holiness and thus, remain "alive" under the corrupt circumstances after the Fall. God foresaw the Fall of His creation, and He created the Sabbath day as a lasting sanctuary where He meets with fallen humanity. He invites us to enter His presence through His rest—the Sabbath Day; He doesn't force us.

By honoring the Sabbath, we are ushered into His presence. The holiness of the Sabbath Day is His presence. Entering God's presence requires personal and communal consecration. (For details on how to consecrate for meeting with God, see p 35). Because God sanctified the Sabbath Day, as we enter into it, we also become sanctified. It is the Lord who makes us holy (Exodus 31:13). He is present in the Sabbath, and when we enter it, His holiness makes us holy.

On Sabbath Day, we reclaim who we are—made in the likeness of God—our authentic state.

The Scripture teaches that once someone or something is dedicated to God through consecration, it becomes holy, and whatever touches any of the holy articles or offerings also becomes holy.

> The sin offering is to be slaughtered before the LORD in the place the burnt offering is slaughtered; it is most holy.... Whatever touches any of the flesh will become holy... (Leviticus 6: 25, 27)
>
> Whatever touches the altar will become holy (Exodus 29:37)

Apostle Paul also teaches this concept in the context of husband and wife.

> For the unbelieving husband has been sanctified through his wife, and the unbelieving wife has been sanctified through her believing husband. (1 Corinthians 7:14)

By entering God's Sabbath, we become holy.

> Moreover, also I gave them my sabbaths, to be a sign between me and them, that they might know that I am the LORD that sanctify them. (Ezekiel 20:12)

God also foresaw humanity's inability to keep His Law, even the Law of the Sabbath. The consequences were deadly.

> The soul that sins is the soul that will die. (Ezekiel 18:20)

The people of the Old Testament, those under the Law, knew and faithfully practiced the true meaning of the Sabbath. Entering the Sabbath Day meant life for them. They experienced "resuscitation" on every Sabbath. Something that died (the soul) during the six days due to sin was revived again on the seventh day. Just like defibrillation in the emergency room resuscitates a cardiac arrest patient, so is the Sabbath, bringing the soul back to life. The Israelites were commanded to come for "resuscitation"—for six days, their spirits would be so engrossed/saturated in corruption that brought death; on the seventh day, they had to be brought back to life. Entering God's holy Sabbath served as "resuscitation" for their souls. Sabbath after Sabbath, life would triumph over death. Sabbath is life under the corrupt circumstances of this fallen world. Humanity is not only refreshed physically when abstaining from physical labor, but is also spiritually resuscitated.

Grace transcends the Old and New Testaments, providing restoration after disobedience to the Law. When entering the Sabbath Day, we return to our initial divine design of purity and holiness. The Sabbath Day provided this opportunity for the people in ancient times and for us today as well.

God "Soulified" the Sabbath

When God created the first six days, He saw that it was good. Five statements attest to God's satisfaction upon creating each day, approving it with "it was good" (Genesis 1). Upon creating humankind, God's approval went up a notch to "very good." Neither of these statements, however, fits the seventh-day quality of creation. God made it holy—a day not equal to anything in the world He created; it was a reality literally "out of this world." What is so special about this day? Everything!

On the sixth day, God imparted His breath of life (נשמת חיים—neshmat haim) into Adam, and he became a living being (נפש חיה—nefesh haya). On the sixth day, God imparted part of Himself, a part He didn't impart into the rest of His creation. In the Hebrew text, the word "life" in the phrase "breath of life" is in the plural form (חיים, haim). The proper translation should be "God... breathed ... the breath of lives" into Adam. The rabbinic discourse on this subject suggests that God breathed into Adam a plurality of life: A soul and a spirit. A similar impartation happened on the Sabbath Day. The Scripture elaborates that "... on the seventh day He rested [שבת, sabbath] and refreshed [וינפש, vainafash].

The Israelites are to observe the Sabbath, celebrating it for the generations to come as a lasting covenant. It will be a sign between me and the Israelites forever, for in six days the LORD made the heavens and the earth, and on the seventh day he rested [שבת, sabbath] and was refreshed [וינפש, vainafash]. (Exodus 31:17)

The Hebrew word for "refresh" is וינפש, vainafash. It shares the same root word as the "breath of life" and "living being" (נפש, nefesh) in Genesis 2:7.

נפש (Genesis 2:7) = **וינפש** (Exodus 31:17) = **נשמת חיים** (Genesis 2:7) = soul

This connection amplifies the meaning of the text in Exodus 31:17, where "refresh" is understood as God re-soulified and re-spirited. God stopped creating and exhaled; He breathed into the Sabbath Day just as He breathed into Adam. God gave the Sabbath a soul; He "soulified" the Sabbath. Sabbath is a Spirit in the form of time[5].

The ancient rabbis taught that for the first six days of the creation, the world had no soul. Only on the seventh day was the world given a soul[6] (וינפש, nefesh=vainafash). Just as Adam became a living being (נפש חיה, nefesh haya) through the breath of God, so the seventh day became "soulified" when God "rested and refreshed" (שבת, sabbath וינפש, vainafash). God refreshed (וינפש, vainafash) on the Sabbath, and the day received a soul (נפש, nefesh).

The Law and the Sabbath

Remember the Sabbath day by keeping it holy. (Exodus 20:8)

The Sabbath is a divine appointment for God's people to meet with God. In the Old Testament times, the entire sacrificial system was designed to prevent spiritual death. The daily temple sacrifices were redemptive sacrifices

5 Heschel, Abraham (2003). The Sabbath. Shambhala, Boston, p. 70

6 Ibid. 77

for remission of sin. They prepared the worshipers to consecrate themselves for the divine meeting on the Sabbath. The mundane of the six days becomes holy on the seventh day.

The appointed Festivals also served the same purpose. Pesah (Passover), Shavuot (Pentecost), Rosh Hashana (New Year), Yom Kippur (Day of Atonement), and Sukkot (Festival of Booths or Tabernacles) were mandated holy assemblies in which God and His people met. Yet, the Sabbath Day was distinct. It surpassed and continues to be elevated to this day in Judaism, above all Festivals; it is considered the most holy day, exalted above all other days.

The Temple law required a special offering for the Sabbath Day (Numbers 28:9,10). It included burnt offerings of two unblemished male lambs, a grain offering, and a drink offering. The burned offering, according to Leviticus 1, and 6:8-13, was an atonement offering. It was required to be entirely burned and symbolized the renewal of fellowship between God and the sinful person. The grain and the drink offerings were part of voluntary thanksgiving offerings, an expression of devotion to God for His goodness and providence. The practice transcends ancient times. Today, the celebration around the table on the Sabbath Day is a similar fellowship gathering of thanksgiving for the goodness of God for His physical and spiritual providence. God's people pray, sing, dance, feast, and delight in God's presence, blessed with the joy of the Lord (Psalms 92; Isaiah 58:13,14).

The Sabbath is an "everlasting ordinance" (Ex 20:11). It is a sign between God and the Israelites forever (Exodus 31:16). The Festivals are not. The Festivals are part of the Law. According to Jesus, the Law will endure until "heaven and earth pass away" (Matthew 5:8). The Sabbath Day precedes the Law of Moses, being blessed and sanctified at the beginning of time, and as the Scripture says, it will be forever, extending into eternity. Sabbath on earth is a glimpse of what eternity is in heaven. The Law has no life in it; the Sabbath has life.

The fourth commandment in the Law of Moses is the command to keep the Sabbath.

> Remember the Sabbath day, to keep it holy. Six days shalt thou labour, and do all thy work: But the seventh day is the sabbath of the LORD thy God: in it thou shalt not do any work, thou, nor thy son, nor thy daughter, thy manservant, nor thy maidservant, nor thy cattle, nor thy stranger that is within thy gates: For in six days the LORD made heaven and earth, the sea, and all that is in them, and rested the seventh day: wherefore the LORD blessed the Sabbath day, and hallowed it. (Exodus 20:8-11)

The instructions are clear,

> Then the LORD said to Moses, "Say to the Israelites, 'You must observe my Sabbaths. This will be a sign between me and you for the generations to come, so you may know that I am the LORD, who makes you holy. Observe the Sabbath, because it is holy to you. Anyone who desecrates it is to be put to death; whoever does any work on that day must be cut off from his people. For six days work is to be done, but the seventh day is a Sabbath of rest, holy to the LORD. Whoever does any work on the Sabbath day is to be put to death. The Israelites are to observe the Sabbath, celebrating it for the generations to come as a lasting covenant. It will be a sign between me and the Israelites forever, for in six days the LORD made the heavens and the earth, and on the seventh day he obtained from work and rested' [refreshed, KJV, NKJV]. (Exodus 31:12-17)

The foreigners were invited to take part in the Sabbath blessing.

> And foreigners who bind themselves to the LORD to minister to him, to love the name of the LORD, and to be

his servants, all who keep the Sabbath without desecrating it and who hold fast to my covenant—these I will bring to my holy mountain and give them joy in my house of prayer. Their burnt offerings and sacrifices will be accepted on my altar; for my house will be called a house of prayer for all nations. (Isaiah 56:6)

Honoring the Sabbath comes with great promise.

"If you keep your feet from breaking the Sabbath and from doing as you please on my holy day, if you call the Sabbath a delight and the LORD's holy day honorable, and if you honor it by not going your own way and not doing as you please or speaking idle words, then you will find your joy in the LORD, and I will cause you to ride in triumph on the heights of the land and to feast on the inheritance of your father Jacob." For the mouth of the LORD has spoken. (Isaiah 58:13,14)

Eternal Sabbath

Jacob was on his way to Paddan Aran to take a wife for himself among the daughters of Laban, his mother's brother. When he reached a certain place on his way to Haran, he stopped for the night because the sun had set. He took one of the stones, put it under his head, and lay down to sleep. He had a dream in which he saw a stairway to heaven. Angels were ascending and descending on it. Above them stood God, who spoke to Jacob, affirming His covenant with him, the same covenant He had made with Jacob's father, Isaac, and his grandfather, Abraham. When Jacob woke up, he was in awe of the encounter. He took the stone he had placed under his head, set it up as a pillar, and poured oil on it. He called the place Bethel, the house of God.

When Jacob awoke from his sleep, he thought, "Surely the Lord is in this place, and I was not aware of it." He was

afraid and said, "How awesome is this place! This is none other than the house of God; this is the gate of heaven."
(Genesis 28:16)

Believers and nonbelievers alike go in and out of the Sabbaths in their lives, not realizing the heavenly treasure of the Sabbath they encounter—God's presence in the Sabbath. Only when we gain the knowledge of the true value of the Sabbath, we, just like Jacob, exclaim, "God is in the Sabbath, and I was not aware of it." Through the knowledge of the Lord's Sabbath, we gain the blessing of the seventh day as intended since the beginning of time. The holiness of the Sabbath sanctifies us.

Psalm 23 ends with the same promise. The Hebrew word translated as "dwell" has the same root as the word "sabbath".

I shall dwell [וְשַׁבְתִּי, vshavti,] in the house of the LORD for ever. (Psalms 23:6)

Thus, ושבתי=שבת; dwell=sabbath. With this understanding, the promise of Psalm 23 resounds with a heavenly appeal, "I shall sabbath (rest) in the house of the LORD for ever." The highest blessing in Psalm 23 is the promise of entering God's rest, His Sabbath, which is His holiness for eternity. Heaven with God is an eternal Sabbath. When Jesus said, "Come to me ... and I will give you rest...", He calls us to enter eternity with Him.

An ancient rabbinic story reveals the spiritual depth of the Sabbath. When God gave the Torah to Israel, He said,

"My children! If you accept the Torah and observe my mitzvot (commandments), I will give you for all eternity a thing most precious that I have in my possession."

"And what is that precious thing which you will give us?" Israel asked.

"The world to come," God responded.

Israel again asked, "Show us in this world an example of the world to come."

"The Sabbath," the Lord replied[7].

The Sabbath is an example of the world to come, the eternity with God in heaven. The world to come is characterized by the kind of holiness possessed by the Sabbath Day only. Sabbath is not only a day but a spiritual state for meeting God. It is a glimpse into eternity with Him.

The Sabbath and the Believers

The author of the Hebrews, in chapters 3 and 4, discusses the subject of the Sabbath Day. The basis of his argument is Psalm 95. The warning from the Lord to the Israelites, in Psalm 95, is stern. The believer is also warned to be aware of hardening of hearts as the Israelites did in the desert when they rebelled against God (Psalms 95:8,9). Their rebellion resulted in them being prevented from entering His rest (sabbath).

> For forty years, I was angry with that generation; I said,
>
> 'They are a people whose hearts go astray, and they have
>
> not known my ways.' So I declared on oath in my anger,
>
> 'They shall never enter my rest.' (Psalms 95:11)

Entering God's rest is an issue of faith and obedience. Without knowing God's way, there is no coming to His Sabbath Day rest. By faith in Jesus, believers enter the Lord's rest.

> For we who have believed enter His rest. (Hebrews 4:3)

Some commentaries identify "rest" in Psalms 95:11 with entering the promised land, where the Israelites will find physical rest from the exhausting battles of their conquest. The author of the Hebrews disagrees with such a conclusion.

> For if Joshua had given them rest, God would not have
>
> spoken later about another day. (Hebrews 4:8)

7 Heschel, Abraham (2003). The Sabbath. Shambhala, Boston, p. 67

By pointing to "another day," the author of the Hebrews refers to the day a believer accepts Christ by faith. That day is the day when the believer enters the Lord's rest. The Sabbath rest is for the people of God.

> There remains, then, a Sabbath-rest for the people of
> God; for anyone who enters God's rest also rests from their
> works, just as God did from his. Let us, therefore, make
> every effort to enter that rest, so that no one will fail by
> following their example of disobedience. (Hebrews 4:9-11)

In Old Testament times, God dwelt in the holy of holies in the Temple. Since the Spirit has been poured on all flesh (Joel 2:28) and since Christ overcame death and restored the immortality of humanity (1 Corinthians 15:54-55), God now dwells within the believer (1 Corinthians 3:16; 6:15). The believer's body is God's temple. No structures can contain the Spirit of God.

And yet, the fourth commandment still stands today as part of the Law of God. Being sanctified at the beginning of time, the Sabbath Day rest continues to contain the holiness of God who sanctified it. Bypassing the Sabbath Day equals bypassing God's presence in the time sanctuary He created for us. Just like Jacob, it is time for the believers to realize that God is in the Sabbath, and we didn't know it.

Church History and the Sabbath Day

Apostle Paul had prophesied that a great apostasy would occur in the Church, resulting in falling away from the truth (2 Thessalonians 2:1-3). Similarly, the Prophet Daniel also prophesied of apostasy,

> And he shall speak great words against the most High, and
> shall wear out the saints of the most High, and think to
> change times and laws: and they shall be given into his
> hand until a time and times and the dividing of time.
> (Daniel 7:25)

From the early church history to this present day, we can see just how these prophecies are being fulfilled. The fourth commandment was altered very early in the history of the Church. Two factors played a significant role. **First**, by the end of the first century AD, the rise of Gnosticism clashed with Christianity. Influenced by philosophers of that age, it sought to reconcile Christianity with Paganism. One of these compromises included the combination of honoring the Lord's day (the first day of the week) and celebrating the day of the Sun. The Romans named the days of the week after the Sun, the Moon, Mars, Mercury, Jupiter, Venus, and Saturn. These were the names of their gods whom they worship on a designated day. Institutionalizing the Sabbath pacified the Sun-day god worshipers. The task was accomplished, first by Emperor Constantine I and later by the Church. In 321 AD, Emperor Constantine I codified Sunday as a day of rest. Christians were already gathering for worship on the Lord's day, and they also honored the sanctity of the Sabbath Day, gathering in synagogues for the same purpose. The Church made the transition official, abolishing the keeping of the Sabbath Day.

The **second** factor was antisemitic by nature. By the third century AD, a strong anti-Jewish sentiment became widespread[8]. The Council of Laodicea in Phrygia Pacatiana (364 AD) responded to these sentiments by codifying the Sunday observance. The Canon 29 officially transferred the solemnity from Saturday to Sunday.

> Christians should not Judaize and should not be idle on the Sabbath, but should work on that day; they should, however, particularly reverence the Lord's day and, if possible, not work on it, as they were Christians[9].

For four centuries after Christ, believers in Yeshua/Jesus were considered a branch of Judaism,[10] just like the Essenes, Pharisees, and Sadducees. Dr.

---

[8] Boyarin, D. (2012) The Jewish Gospels: The Story of the Jewish Christ. The New Press, New York, p. 15

[9] https://www.newadvent.org/fathers/3806.htm

[10] Boyarin, D. (2012) The Jewish Gospels: The Story of the Jewish Christ. The New Press, New York, p. 13

Boyarin provides evidence that the first Church was Jewish, despite having a large Gentile presence, because it adhered to the core Jewish beliefs and observances.

Fifteen centuries later, Protestantism didn't reverse the practice enforced by the Council of Laodicea, as it was already deeply entrenched in the social customs, and Sunday worship was universally observed. They have continued the practice even though it rests upon the authority of the Fourth-century Church and not upon the Holy Scriptures. Tradition was inserted as Law.

The Scripture, however, is consistent in affirming the sanctity of the Sabbath Day. It transcends the Old and New Testaments. The Jerusalem council, around 48-50AD, (Acts 15) confirms this fact. The apostles never discussed the issue of the Sabbath. It was neither controversial for the Jews nor for the Gentiles. The Sabbath Day was observed universally by all believers across cultures. The apostles called the meeting to discuss the question of circumcision (Acts 15:6), not the question of whether or not the Sabbath observance should continue. The council sent a letter to the churches in Antioch, Syria, and Cilicia (Acts 15:23-29), with their decision. It stated,

> You are to abstain from food sacrificed to idols, from blood, from the meat of strangled animals, and from sexual immorality. You will do well to avoid these things. (Acts 15:29).

No mention of abolishing the Sabbath! Our forefathers of the faith, the apostles, affirmed the Sabbath Day as our spiritual heritage.

Furthermore, there is no biblical reference for communal worship on the Sabbath Day. Instead, every family celebrated the Day of Rest on their own as the Law of Moses commanded.

> Bear in mind that the Lord has given you the Sabbath; that is why on the sixth day he gives you bread for two days. Everyone is to stay where they are on the seventh day; no one is to go out. (Exodus 16:29)

The local synagogue with the Sabbath liturgy started about a century before Christ. It was a new Jewish organization not operated by priests but by laymen. The synagogue was a response to Antiochus Epiphanes' persecution of the Jews. He desecrated the Second Temple by sacrificing a pig on the altar and outlawing the Jewish laws and observances. The synagogue became an alternative to the Temple, especially after the destruction of the Second Temple and the dispersion of the Jewish people. Jesus went to the synagogue on the Sabbath Day, but to the temple on the Jewish festivals.

CONCLUSION

Sabbath is rest. There is no scriptural mandate for communal worship; it is a family celebration with fine dining and joy as we enter the Lord's holy time sanctuary for fellowship with Him. When we consecrate ourselves for the Sabbath Day, we enter God's holiness, and we are sanctified. This is our heritage, and if it is not claimed, we miss its spiritual endowment. Just like Jacob, one day, we would realize that God is in the Sabbath and we didn't know it. The Letter to the Hebrews, however, gives us consolation that through Christ, the believer is now endowed with the same holiness, regardless of the day of the week.

When believers enter the Sabbath Day, they enter God's eternal holy presence as ordained since the beginning of time. When believers gather for Sunday worship (or any other day), their holiness evokes God's holy presence, and their assembly makes the day holy. Sunday has no holiness of its own; the Sabbath Day has. On the Sabbath, the believers enter the Sabbath Day to meet with God, but on Sunday, Jesus enters the day to meet with the believers, just as He promised.

> For where two or three are gathered together in my name,
> there am I in the midst of them. (Matthew 18:20)

Jesus is in the Sabbath Day; He is the Lord of the Sabbath (Matthew 12:8). He made and blessed the Sabbath Day for humankind, a day when we meet with Him and rest in His presence. Again, we enter His Sabbath to meet Jesus, but Jesus enters Sunday (or any other day) to meet with us when we gather in His name.

From an eternal perspective, Sunday as a time frame would cease to exist. Saturday, as a holy sanctuary of God, however, passes into eternity. Should, then, the believers keep the Sabbath Day once they become aware of its eternal spiritual benefits? Why not? The gain is great: A double dip in the holy presence of God. Jesus continues to call us today to enter His rest and be sanctified by the holiness of the Sabbath Day.

"Come to me, all you who are weary and burdened, and I

will give you rest." (Matthew 11:28-30)

EHAD with GOD

REFLECTION—Week Six

Reflection 1: Give Him Five (5 minutes)— a daily practice of God's presence (see description on pages 41 and 63 under "Deep calls to deep" section)

Reflection 2: Daily confession and repentance in prayer to Christ—our high priest; crucify the flesh, wash with the blood, fill with the Holy Spirit (page 13)

Reflection 3: God's Healing

God's Healing

Task: The texts below describe stories of healing as part of Jesus' ministry. Note the differences in the attitude of heart the people exhibited. Discuss your thoughts and the lessons you learned.

Healing at the Pool of Bethesda (John 5:1-7)

Sometime later, Jesus went up to Jerusalem for a Feast of the Jews. Now there is in Jerusalem near the Sheep Gate a pool, which in Aramaic is called Bethesda and which is surrounded by five covered colonnades. Here, a great number of disabled people used to lie—the blind, the lame, the paralyzed. One who was there had been an invalid for thirty-eight years. When Jesus saw him lying there and learned that he had been in this condition for a long time, he asked him, "Do you want to get well?"

"Sir," the invalid replied, "I have no one to help me into the pool when the water is stirred. While I am trying to get in, someone else goes down ahead of me."

Then Jesus said to him, "Get up! Pick up your mat and walk." At once the man was cured; he picked up his mat and walked. The day on which this took place was a Sabbath, and so the Jewish leaders said to the man who had been healed, "It is the Sabbath; the law forbids you to carry your mat." But he replied, "The man who made me well said to me, 'Pick up your mat and walk' " (John 5:1-7).

Healing at the Mountainside (Matthew 15:29–31)

Jesus left there and went along the Sea of Galilee. Then he went up on a mountainside and sat down. Great crowds came to him, bringing the lame, the blind, the crippled, the mute and many others, and laid them at his feet; and he healed them. The people were amazed when they saw the mute speaking, the crippled made well, the lame walking and the blind seeing. And they praised the God of Israel (Matthew 15:29–31).

Healing the Man with Leprosy (Matthew 8:1-4)

When Jesus came down from the mountainside, large crowds followed him. A man with leprosy came and knelt before him and said, "Lord, if you are willing, you can make me clean." Jesus reached out his hand and touched the man. "I am willing," he said. "Be clean!" Immediately he was cleansed of his leprosy. Then Jesus said to him, "See that you don't tell anyone. But go, show yourself to the priest and offer the gift Moses commanded, as a testimony to them" (Matthew 8:1-4).

Discussion

When Jesus entered the courts of the pool of Bethesda He did not heal everyone who was present at that moment. He could have easily done that. Out of the many sick individuals around the pool, He approached and healed only one! Did He not have compassion on all of them? The issue here is not a lack of compassion; no other heart bled for us with greater compassion for humanity than His. Jesus delivered the Father's will for that one suffering man at that particular time. Only that man, at the pool, on that day, was ready to receive his healing. God, who sees into that man's heart, saw his readiness and ministered to him by healing him.

When the Lord heals, He restores the health of the whole person. The man's physical healing was seen immediately by many, but there was a much greater healing accomplished in his heart that was seen only by Jesus. For this reason, after the healing, Jesus found the man at the Temple and said to him, "See, you are well again. Stop sinning or something worse may happen to you" (John 5:14). What is the "worst" that could happen to the man? The man knew what Jesus meant because he knew the Word of God.

The soul who sins is the one who will die. (Ezekiel 18:4b)

Jesus warned the man of the detrimental consequences of sin in his life. As it was then with the ill man at the Bethesda pool, so it is with us now. God alone renders the timing, the form, and the delivery of God's healing provision. We must be ready, spiritually cleansed, for His healing.

In the time of my favor, I will answer you, and in the day of salvation, I will help you. (Isaiah 49:8)

In contrast to the healing at the Bethesda pool are the healings on the mountainside and the leper. While Jesus healed only one man at the pool, Scripture tells us that He healed everyone brought to Him on the mountainside (Matthew 4:24). The number of healings is not the only difference in these two cases but in the attitudes of the heart as well. The first was an attitude of waiting and wailing; the second was an attitude of actively seeking and finding. God deals with us differently when we approach Him wholeheartedly with our problems. The Lord desires to make His will known to His children and waits for us to acknowledge His sovereignty. Approaching God is an important step that puts us in the correct position to lay our requests before Him. Like the father who did not run after his prodigal son but waited for him, so is God waiting with outstretched arms for us, His children, to return and acknowledge Him, to acknowledge His healing power. Throughout the Scripture, God repeatedly calls for closeness with Him. God told Moses, upon giving the Law,

"Come up to me on the mountain" (Exodus 24:12; Deuteronomy 10:1). God repeatedly called the Israelites, through the prophets, to make peace with Him. Jesus instructed us to be active.

> Ask and it will be given to you; seek and you will find; knock and the door will be opened to you. For everyone who asks receives; he who seeks finds; and to him who knocks, the door will be opened. (Matthew 7:7-8)

Our coming to God is a conscious choice based on our free will. It shows the readiness of the mind and heart to seek God first. In the spiritual realm, such choice places us as receivers of God's grace and mercy. It displays obedience to the first commandment: "Love the LORD your God with all your heart and with all your soul and with all your strength" (Deuteronomy 6:5).

According to Jeremiah 29:11-14, our attitude should be:

1. "You will call upon me and come and pray to me," (v.12)

2. "and I will listen to you" (v.12)

3. The third point is a specific condition to the first two. "You will seek me and find me when you seek me with all your heart. I will be found by you" (v. 13-14)

Question: Tell us your story of healing. How does it compare with the ill man at Bethesda pool, the leper, and the people who followed Jesus at the mountainside?

_____

_____

_____

_____

_____

_____

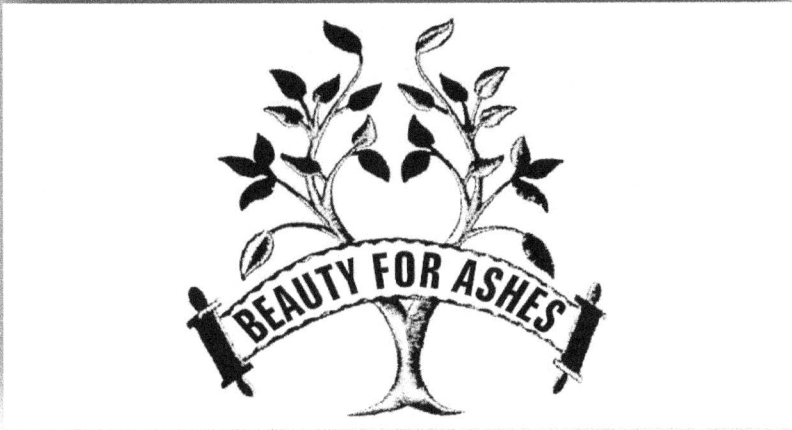

SESSION SEVEN

SHAME AND GUILT, BETRAYAL AND TRUST

Shame and Guilt

Shame is the fear of exposure. Embarrassment is not shame. Often, these two are used interchangeably, but each leaves a distinctive "dent" on the soul. Falling short while performing mundane tasks can be embarrassing, and depending on the "thickness of one's skin," it might or might not leave an emotional scar. There are no detrimental consequences to the state of mind and heart. This is the "dent" of embarrassment.

Shame, on the other hand, is a deeply seeded fear that our words, behaviors, facial expressions, and body language might reveal past wounds (dents) of the heart. Flawed character exposure or admission of behavior disapproved by societal standards is traumatic and deeply shameful. Shame forces us to build tall, impenetrable walls around ourselves. Shame circumvents ethics to keep "prying eyes" at arm's length. Shame is skillful in displaying a polished image and spends a tremendous amount of energy to ensure that the discrepancies between one's public and one's true self are never discovered.

Shame puts up a veneer-tin facade that might seem strong in public but crumbles at one's deaf-silent, lonely corner. Shame dreads exposure of self. Shame has acquired all the above coping mechanisms to remain a secret. Shame is a drain on the body, the soul, and the spirit. Shame is exhausting. When exposed, shame might cause such unbearable pain that it could shrink the soul away from the joys of life. Shame is the uttermost depravity. Shame is the lifeline of trauma.

Figure 1.

SHAME	GUILT
I am a bad person. I am worthless. I am unlovable, broken.	I did something bad.

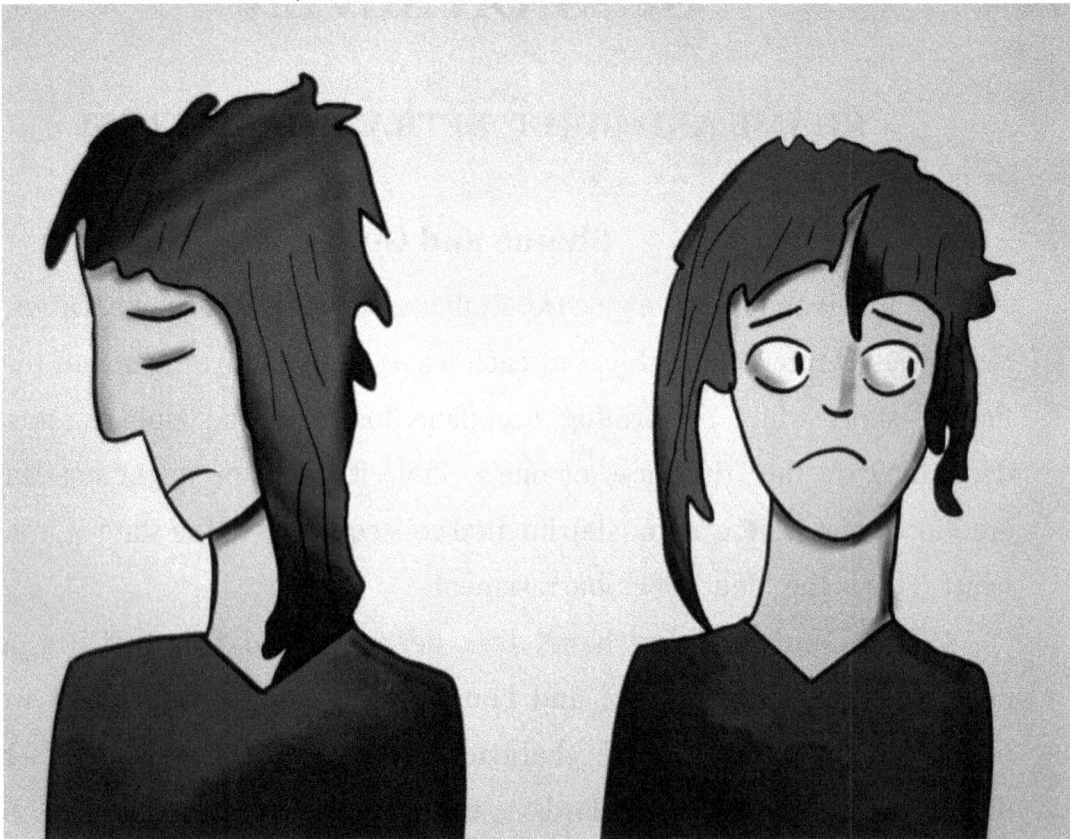

Question: Think of actions and situations that you feel ashamed about. What would you rather hide when you tell your story of trauma?

_____

_____

Task: Rate the following statements (1 means "not at all true", 10 means "completely true").

I love myself

1	2	3	4	5	6	7	8	9	10
◯	◯	◯	◯	◯	◯	◯	◯	◯	◯

People like me

1	2	3	4	5	6	7	8	9	10
◯	◯	◯	◯	◯	◯	◯	◯	◯	◯

People listen to what I have to say

1	2	3	4	5	6	7	8	9	10
◯	◯	◯	◯	◯	◯	◯	◯	◯	◯

I am not a bad person

1	2	3	4	5	6	7	8	9	10
◯	◯	◯	◯	◯	◯	◯	◯	◯	◯

Shame and self-esteem have a negative correlation. The higher the degree of shame, the lower the self-esteem. The above self-evaluation prompts help reveal the degree to which shame has a stronghold on your spiritual health.

Shame is a practice of the flesh. We deal with shame as we deal with any other practice of the flesh—we repent from it and crucify it on the cross of Jesus (detailed description in section six).

Manifestations of Shame

We might successfully hide shame from people, even from our immediate family, but we cannot hide the contents of our hearts from God. Many don't consider shame detrimental to their walk with God and don't put too much weight on the impact of shame on the human soul. After all, it is not murder, adultery, theft, or idolatry, or among the seven deadly sins. Yet shame is the very first sin manifested immediately after the Fall. Scripture reports the story of shame in Genesis 3:8-21, depicting two distinct manifestations.

Concealment—Adam and Eve hid from God. They wanted to conceal their disobedience, but contrary to their efforts, their shame was quickly exposed; it has been paraded before humanity since the Scripture recorded it.

Defensiveness—Adam and Eve had identical reactions to exposure to sin. Instead of taking full responsibility for their actions, they blamed others for their choices. They became defensive.

The story of Adam and Eve is a shared story of all humanity. As we point at the speck of Adam and Eve, can we see the log in our own eyes (Matthew 5:7)? Yes, we are also guilty and plagued by the same kind of shame. When confronted with our sins of disobedience, we become defensive, covering our tracks, deflecting the truth, and rejecting accountability. Justifying one's actions does not secure justification in the eyes of God. It only becomes a display of reckless trespassing. Have you ever wondered whether the course of human history would have differed had Adam and Eve confessed and repented instead of blaming others for their failure? We might still be in the Garden of Eden.

Good is Evil and Evil is Good

Today, in post-modern society, the freedom of expression asserts the eradication of shame. Religious morality is cast away as old-fashioned biblical ethos. This is the old Garden of Eden rebellion, repudiating sinful behaviors as shameful. The removal of biblical laws removes the societal moral compass: Everyone is doing what is right in their own eyes (Judges 17:6). From this perspective, sin is not only tolerated but highly celebrated. Thus, these behaviors grant the person a great status and acknowledgment instead of shame. Once shameful and secretive behaviors are now proudly flaunted to the world, and people who practice them are exemplified as role models.

The contemptible twisting of the spiritual reality to fit one's own "truths" doesn't change God's reality and His eternal Truth. It is a blunt naiveté to believe that our rebellion will ever affect the Almighty God who was, is, and will be for all eternity. Denial of God is a blindness of the soul. The Scripture reveals God, who is omnipotent, omnipresent, and omniscient.

> For this is what the high and exalted One says—he who lives forever, whose name is holy: "I live in a high and holy place, but also with the one who is contrite and lowly in spirit, to revive the spirit of the lowly and to revive the heart of the contrite." (Isaiah 57:15)
>
> From heaven the LORD looks down and sees all mankind; from his dwelling place he watches all who live on earth—he who forms the hearts of all, who considers everything they do. (Psalms 33:13-15)
>
> "Who can hide in secret places so that I cannot see them?" declares the LORD. "Do not I fill heaven and earth?" declares the LORD. (Jeremiah 23:24)

God, through the Prophet Isaiah, condemned the state of today's abominable celebration of shameful practices.

> Woe to those who call evil good and good evil, who put darkness for light and light for darkness, who put bitter for sweet and sweet for bitter. (Isaiah 5:20)

We are called to love what is good and hate what is evil (Romans 12:9). Practices inconsistent with the Kingdom of God are evil. When sin becomes accepted and widely practiced in a society, it loses its appeal for judgment. This was valid for the people from the Prophet Jeremiah's time, and it is valid for our own time today.

> 'Are they ashamed of their loathsome conduct? No, they have no shame at all; they do not even know how to blush. So they will fall among the fallen; they will be brought down when I punish them,' says the LORD. (Jeremiah 6:15)

In the Prophet Jeremiah's time, God's people had gotten so accustomed to sin that they no longer felt guilty for engaging in those practices. So are we today. Shame is evidence of a working conscience. Shame is the "godly sorrow" that encourages repentance and leads to salvation (2 Corinthians 7:8-10). Ignoring the sense of shame and continuing in sinful practices will eventually lead one to be "seared in their conscience" and no longer be ashamed (1 Timothy 4:2). It is a deafness to the call of the Holy Spirit to run away from danger and death. It becomes one's self-warranted destruction.

Regaining Dignity—Healing From Shame

Unresolved traumas from sexual violence and sexually deviant behaviors are death threats to the soul, stamping individuals with a deep sense of shame. The scarring from these particular origins of shame forms a state of depravity— an existence that shrinks the soul back from life. It is the opposite of the state of dignity—the divine image in which God created humankind at the beginning of time. Healing from such traumatic events requires the restoration of lost dignity. One must extend genuine repentance and subsequent forgiveness toward the perpetrator.

Depravity and dignity are two warring forces, and depending on which one has the upper hand, it determines the health of the psyche. It is like the dichotomy we face when commanded to "love your enemies" (Matthew 5:38) and to "hate what is evil and cling to what is good" (Romans 12:9). The victims of violence face an impossible task: While instructed to hate the evil they endured, they must, at the same time, love their enemy, even the perpetrator.

There are two responses to this humanly impossible task. The first response accounts for those individuals relying on their strength of character and determination to forgive and "love" the perpetrator-enemy. They display a nice attitude, avoiding tensions and conflicts. However, this is the self-preservation mechanism of numbing feelings. Once the seed of soul-numbing is sown, it reaps an abundant harvest of maladaptive behaviors. While functioning within the predictable patterns of life, these individuals feel safe. The threat comes from those unpredictable circumstances that pose continuous stress over the individual. Then, despite the effort to conceal what is inside, the pain erupts from within like a volcano of anger, contempt, and hatred. Jesus described these outbursts as an illness of the soul.

> Out of the overflow of the heart, the mouth speaks. (Matthew
> 12:34)

The case of Rose (page 94) exemplifies this spiritual condition. The silly tug of a hanger triggered a disproportionate response that revealed the true condition of the other woman's heart. The hanger didn't cause her pain; the old, unresolved trauma did.

The second response is the total reliance on the healing power of Jesus. This is the way of healing through becoming EHAD with God—the healing approach to trauma first introduced in session one and then in much greater detail in session six.

The Guilt: Self-Condemnation—The Inability to Forgive Oneself

Guilt is a killer. It squeezes the joy of a believer's life. Life to the fullest (John 10:10) seems unattainable. It is just an existence on life support fueled by the practice of self-denial and self-punishment. Scripture is memorized without being internalized. Good deeds are "dead deeds" because they are self-redemptive deeds. Working hard for God is just a payback for the sins of the past. This is the sorrowful existence of self-condemnation, the inability to forgive oneself.

Spiritual laws, however, contain no such self-redemptive postulations. No one can pay or self-redeem for past wrongdoings. Only God can atone for them. And He did, once and for all, on the cross. No matter how grievous, all sins have been nailed to the cross and paid for. They have been forgiven; they have been whited out. From God's eternal perspective, they don't exist. Once forgiven, they are forgiven into eternity. The Book of Life (Revelation 12:27) doesn't contain them. They are erased from God's memories. For many believers, however, the reality is tormenting: Their memories continue to afflict the soul. Many continue to agonize over past offenses, carrying their burden, even though they have already been forgiven. This is the enemy's most effective weapon. If the Devil cannot get a believer through seduction, manipulations, and lies, he resorts to guilt. He augments its significance by relentlessly pounding it on the believer's consciousness. It is a big, fat lie out of the pit of hell. No such thing exists. We only lose this battle if we agree with the enemy. Every believer knows and often quotes Apostle Paul's words of assurance that "There is no condemnation for those who are in Christ Jesus" (Romans 8:1). And yet, we fail to live up to that truth. Being unable to accept God's forgiveness is an impediment for many believers to their relationship with God. This inner conflict must be resolved; otherwise, if left unattended, it brings God's judgment on the guilt-laden person. God, who is sovereign in His just judgments and has ultimately forgiven the sins, is now undermined by our subjective feelings. It's not a good position to find yourself in before the Eternal God. Indeed, this is a dreadful position. The Law of God postulates that we should forgive because we have been forgiven (Matthew 6:12). The command to forgive also extends forgiveness towards oneself. Who are we to withhold forgiveness when God has already forgiven? Withholding forgiveness towards oneself is a trespass in itself. The guilt can only be removed by confronting and rejecting the enemy's lie. Deal with guilt as with any other practice of the flesh: Confess, repent, and crucify it on the cross of Jesus. The memories of the offense will always be there, but the debilitating burden of guilt will be gone. This is the freedom from guilt.

Prayer for Rejection of Guilt

Jesus, I confess that guilt plagues me. I have accepted your forgiveness, yet I admit that I continue to carry the guilt of my sins. I now recognize that the enemy has manipulated me and has kept me captive to a lie. Forgive me, Jesus, for allowing the enemy to succeed in his deception. Now, I take the sin of guilt —the inability to forgive myself—and nail it to the cross. I declare it dead on the cross. I claim the cleansing power of your blood, spilled on the cross to wash me clean. I call upon your Spirit of Life to come and reside in me. May my guilt be replaced with Your peace. In Jesus' name, I pray for freedom from guilt. Amen!

Now, write on a piece of paper with large letters and post it in a prominent place in your home the following statement:

NO GUILT IN LIFE, NO FEAR IN DEATH[11]

Keep the postings for at least a week as you pray the above prayer so that the mind agrees with the heart that this is God's ultimate truth.

Powerlessness and Ambivalence

Jesus told them another parable: "The kingdom of heaven is like a man who sowed good seed in his field. But while everyone was sleeping, his enemy came and sowed weeds among the wheat, and went away. When the wheat sprouted and formed heads, then the weeds also appeared." The

---

[11] A line from the hymn "In Christ Alone" by Keith Getty and Stuart Townend, 2001

owner's servants came to him and said, 'Sir, didn't you sow good seed in your field? Where then did the weeds come from?' " 'An enemy did this,' he replied.' " The servants asked him, 'Do you want us to go and pull them up?' " 'No,' he answered, 'because while you are pulling the weeds, you may uproot the wheat with them. Let both grow together until the harvest. At that time I will tell the harvesters: First collect the weeds and tie them in bundles to be burned; then gather the wheat and bring it into my barn.' "

(Matthew 13: 24-30)

Every child coming into this world is a blessing. Their soul is like a fertile field where God has planted good seeds for abundant life. And yet, being born into a world seeded with violence, immorality, and corruption, it is inevitable that these seeds will simultaneously be sown into the innocent ground of the child's soul, as well. As the child grows, these two kinds of seeds grow and mature also, yielding a harvest of wheat and weed. Jesus said, "Let both grow together until the harvest" (v.30). He further instructed that the weeds be collected first for the fire and then the good wheat to be brought into His barn.

The *EHAD with GOD* approach to healing follows Christ's instructions. The strategy is to identify the weeds, pull them out, and cast them away, "burn them," as Jesus said. Once they are removed, the remaining harvest will be seen for what it is: A good seed that produced a good harvest—a pure and beautiful soul destined to God's eternal barns—the Kingdom of God.

The road to healing is like plucking out the bad weeds from a beautiful garden. We have uprooted the weeds of anger, hatred, resentment, bitterness, and unforgiveness. Those are weeds that, if not uprooted on time, can grow into tree-like structures that would later need special equipment to cut down and destroy. Indeed, if you have followed the instructions of *EHAD with GOD*, you have now cut them down and removed them. The soul suffocated under the weed invasion is now rejoicing in the Son-lit freedom. At this point on the narrow road, we are ready to deal with those "smaller" weeds, which have the appearance of a nice ground cover, but in reality, they suck the lifeblood out of the field—the soul. These are the weeds of powerlessness and ambivalence.

Powerlessness

Powerlessness is the act of robbing an individual of the right to choose. Free will is divinely granted by God. It is the sovereign right to make conscious decisions about oneself. When this right is violated, it sinks the soul into utter depravity. This is the seed of powerlessness.

The powerlessness stems from the fact that the victim had no way to change the situation. In the case of abuse, the perpetrator blocks any attempt at a change of circumstances, leaving no chance of escape. A child who is born into an abusive family situation doesn't understand its depravity; the child accepts it as a part of life. Complying with the abuser's demands is a survival mechanism.

Note: The content for the rest of the session is primarily relevant to victims of sexual abuse and human trafficking.

When sexual abuse comes with consistent attention with gifts, love, and pleasure, sexual acts are viewed as part of the way of life through which one expresses affection. Later in life, this experience codifies the understanding that a sexual act is an imminent, natural part of all personal encounters. The sanctity of sexual purity is a foreign concept. The deep longing for love and acceptance is coupled with the duty and the desire always to provide sexual favors. This is the ugly beast of being born into promiscuity. At this point, the abuser had robbed the victim twice: Once of choice and once of dignity.

When the sexual encounter comes with pain and violence, the dynamics are entirely different. It is not love, affection, and pleasure that keep the victim silent, but the mortal fear of more pain and violence. The terror is shrouded in secrecy. The compliance is secured with treats. This is an act of quadruple aggravation upon an individual's physical, mental, emotional, and spiritual faculties. In contrast to the "pleasure" abuse that leads to promiscuity, this experience throws the victim into "shutting down" mode, which postulates not only complete avoidance of any future sexual encounters but also complete avoidance of individuals from the gender associated with the sexual abuse. The above-described situations of child sexual abuse result in ambivalence of the responses.

Ambivalence

Ambivalence represents the tension of having simultaneously opposite and contradictory attitudes or feelings toward a person. In the same breath, one may experience attraction and repulsion. Physical sensations of sexual pleasure are juxtaposed against the grave violation of personhood. Pleasure augments the pangs of guilt and shame. This is the seed of ambivalence.

Prolonged exposure to abuse shrinks the soul. The damage is irreversible. What was done cannot be undone. What eyes have seen cannot be unseen. What the ears have heard cannot be unheard. The stamp of abuse on the soul dents the character; it distorts perceptions and contaminates relationships. This is the lonely corner of powerlessness. From that perspective, the world is a hostile place, and the sinking of the soul seems an inevitable alternative to life. Powerlessness breeds despair; it is a life without light, moving forward without advancing.

There is, however, a way out of this nothingness, as simple as a child's world of fairytales. As children believe in incredible fairytale stories, we are invited to become just like children and accept God's redemptive story of humanity narrated in the Bible. It speaks of washing, cleansing, and purifying through the blood of Jesus and a renewal of life beyond anything one has ever imagined. Indeed, this is not a fairytale; this is the unseen reality of God. It promises a complete renewal of body, soul, and spirit. The only condition for this amazing transformation is to believe the old Calvary story: He is God Almighty who died in my stead to redeem me from the punishment of death for my sins. He was buried and rose on the third day to eternal life so I can enter eternity with Him. This is God's provision for a second chance in life. At this point, a completely new life. The new life is now aligned with God's divine design, as it was intended from the beginning of time.

This is God's gift. As we walk on the narrow road towards eternity with Christ, we are miraculously transformed from "glory to glory" into His image (2 Corinthians 3:18). We shed our old nature with its corrupted character traits and are clothed with His divine nature. Thus, His purity becomes our purity. It is a spiritual law that postulates that once the person believes in Christ as Lord, God, and Savior, all is new. The new nature of Christ Himself now replaces the old self. The dents in the character, the distorted perceptions of the mind, and the contaminated patterns of our relationships are all redeemed. Under these new conditions, His wisdom becomes our wisdom; His holiness—our holiness; His beauty—our beauty. Everyone can be redeemed; everyone can be washed, purified, and sanctified. The biggest sinner can become an oak of righteousness —a planting of the Lord for the display of His splendor (Isaiah 61:3).

The Story of Lila

I was born into a happy family and grew up as a happy little girl. I was showered with special attention that kept telling me I was the most beautiful and loved girl in the universe. My mom said that when I was born, a word traveled fast through the maternity ward of a beautiful baby being just born. All hospital staff streamed through the room, desiring to see this unusual beauty. I knew I was special.

My family is affectionate. We hug and kiss, and little kids are cuddled in adults' arms for comfort, love, and protection. I remember the sheer strength of my dad's strong arms, lifting me and swirling me up in the air. I never, even for a moment, doubted that these strong arms would always be there for me to land safely. I giggled and screamed with excitement, not with fear. I trusted my dad also when, one day, he said that I was a big girl now and that he would show me his love in a special new way. He said it would be our special love secret. I immediately liked it very much. The touch and the kisses all came with lavished gifts, candies, and words of love. And I responded with love as well. I loved my dad, and it was good to see how our love game made him so happy.

My mom was a dentist, working long hours, but my dad was with me. For our extended family and friends, we were still the affectionate family we have always been.

Years passed as I grew older, and so did my beauty. The boys in school were falling heads over heels for me. They competed to impress me, and I loved the attention. Very early, they began to touch me the same way my dad did. And it felt equally pleasant. I loved them back, reciprocating the pleasure they showered me with.

I went through middle school, constantly hearing derogatory remarks hurled at me. "They are just jealous that boys like me," I concluded and became more determined, clinging to the only way I knew to get attention, affection, and love.

The day I fell in love changed my life forever. It was different for me, but not for him. I wanted more of him, but it was not mutual. He only spoke to me when away from prying eyes. In public, he pretended not to know me. Pain pierced my heart. There was a grievous irony projected over my very young life: Knowing how to "love" didn't secure the winning of my first true love. But I was a survivor. I shut my heart down, drowning the pain. I forced myself to move on, trying to fill the longing inside with more infamous sexual experiences. Sex became just the good food that satisfied my sexual appetites, which, on its terms, extinguished the flames of my first love.

Task: How can you help Lila heal from the childhood sexual trauma? Lead her on the way of the cross for healing through sanctification in Christ.

_____

_____

_____

_____

Betrayal and Trust

Betrayal is universal. No one escapes its ugly reality, and no one is insured against it. It is the human inability to stay on the apparent path of YES or NO (Matthew 5:37). Everything else is a betrayal. Betrayal scars souls, kills spirits, distorts relationships, and leaves the person with a marred worldview where hypocrisy and manipulations of circumstance are the norm, not the exception.

The responses to a betrayal are on a continuum, with a low end of forgive and forget to a high end of hatred, rage, and vengeance, from feeling bad to developing Post Traumatic Stress Disorder (PTSD). Believers who have gone through traumatic events are prone to experience intense reactions to betrayals with high-end responses. When the victims are children, and the perpetrator is a parent, the betrayal is off the common scale. It is an occurrence of its own proportions. It is the ultimate distortion of family relationships with maximum damage to the child. It is a new form of ugly and a new shape of evil that falls into its own category. This kind of betrayal is not a "natural" occurrence. Only the existence of "spiritual forces of evil in the heavenly realms" (Ephesians 6:12) can explain this evil.

Rebuilding trust after betrayal is a lifelong endeavor. The success of regaining trust depends on the severity of the trauma and the consequential development of possible PTSD. Survivors of physical, emotional, and sexual abuse may experience more complex struggles because of the nature of the abuse, especially when the victim is a minor.

Trust is an inborn disposition toward life, which has been divinely imparted since the beginning of time. Every betrayal diminishes trust, and the consistency of met expectations strengthens it. Either tendency forms very early in childhood and determines the forms of attachment an individual develops as an adult. These styles of attachment become permanent personality traits.

John Bowlby (1907-1990), a child psychiatrist, developed the theory of attachment styles. He found patterns in the formation of psychological connectedness in early child-parent relationships. The earliest bonds formed by children with their caregivers determine their capacity to trust later in life. Based on this understanding, there are four attachment types: Secure, anxious, avoidant, and disorganized (fearful). Later in life, these childhood attachment styles become part of the adult personality. There are three major adult attachment styles, proceeding from attachment types formed in early childhood: Secure, anxious, and ambivalent. (See Table 2.)

Secure attachment: Children with a secure attachment pattern show moderate distress when the caregiver leaves but can quickly compose themselves when the caregiver returns. Such children feel protected by their attachment figures and trust that the caregiver will return. In adults, this attachment style represents a low fear of failure and a high need for achievement. Such individuals are skillful at conflict resolution in relationships; they avoid manipulation, are comfortable with intimacy, and forgive quickly.

Avoidant attachment: There are two variants under this category. Adults with dismissive-avoidant attachment styles appear distant, avoiding attachment altogether. They desire a high level of independence and view themselves as self-sufficient. They tend to have a low opinion of people they perceive as dependent on them. They deal with conflict by distancing themselves from the situation that caused it.

Adults with an anxious-avoidant attachment style have mixed feelings and mixed needs regarding romantic relationships. They desire emotional closeness and intimacy but feel uncomfortable when they have it. Such individuals tend to be pessimistic, having a less pleasant outlook on life. They suppress their feelings and avoid dealing with conflicts. They are seen as loners, but inwardly, they crave intimacy.

Table 2. Adult Attachment Style Based on Type of Attachment Formed in Infancy[12]

DISPLAYED CHARACTERISTICS

ATTACHMENT STYLES	AS A CHILD	AS AN ADULT
SECURE	Able to separate from parent	Have trusting lasting relationships
	Seek comfort from parents when frightened	Tend to have good self-esteem
	Return of parents is met with positive emotions	Comfortable sharing feelings with friends and partners
	Prefer parents to strangers	Seek out social support
AVOIDANT	May avoid parents	May have problems with intimacy
	Don't seek much comfort or contact from parents	Invest little emotion in social and romantic relationships
	Show little or no preference between parent and stranger	Unable or unwilling to share thoughts and feelings with others
AMBIVALENT	May be wary of strangers	Reluctant to become close to others
	Become distressed when parents leave	Worry that partner doesn't love them
	Not comforted by the return of the parent	Very distraught when a relationship ends

Ambivalent attachment: Adults with this attachment style desire closeness and intimacy and often become overly dependent on their partners. These individuals have less favorable views about themselves and their partners. They are typically less trusting and more emotionally expressive,

---

[12] https://www.heartspringtherapy.ca/post/attachment-styles-and-adult-relatonships

borderline neurotic. Incessant cycles of love and hate are the drama they create in relationships. They are unstable, less predictable, and trusting no one.

Any form of child abuse distorts the character and results in the formation of maladaptive behaviors later in life. It affects perceptions, relationships, and ethics. The *EHAD with GOD* methodology, when applied diligently, successfully addresses the above issues, leading to positive changes and the ultimate healing of maladaptive patterns of behavior.

Task: Identify your adult attachment style. Reflect on how childhood upbringing and possible traumatic events have shaped your adult character.

_____
_____
_____
_____
_____
_____
_____
_____
_____
_____
_____
_____
_____
_____
_____
_____
_____
_____
_____
_____
_____

The Power of The Dog—Biblical References of Betrayal

December 2021

It was again that time of the year when the bright lights outside rivaled Mary's bright contentment of heart inside—her true light of Christmas. It would be a quiet evening for Mary. Her husband and son were part of the cast presenting the live Christmas story—a yearly event organized by their church in Burnet, Texas. Thousands of out-of-town visitors would descend back in time, walking the streets of the ancient Bethlehem village, and be visually stimulated to experience the old Christmas story.

Back at home, the void of noise and clatter suddenly made the house seem too small to contain the steadily expanding wall-to-wall silence. Mary clicked the TV receiver, and the bright light immediately dispersed silence and loneliness. The Netflix screen opened, and her attention zeroed in on a title that conveyed cowboy entertainment: The Power of the Dog. The lead actor's name was decisive for her choice—Benedict Cumberbatch. With increasing anticipation, she was engulfed by the developing plot that transported her back a century to 1925 Montana. It was a story of trust and betrayal. Later into the night, Mary's mind lingered on the unexpected twist. A rude and inconsiderate man extended his hand for reconciliation to a fragile and timid youth he had offended earlier. Despite the problems in their relationship, they shook hands in mutual agreement to forgive and accept. This notion, however, was deceptive. The apparent reconciliation was a strategic move for the youth, giving him closer access to his target to plan and execute his revenge. The story ended tragically. The complete trust of the "rude" character met the betrayal of the "proper" character, causing the one who trusted the new relationship to his ultimate demise.

Mary lingered on the story late into the night. She sympathized with the main character, who tried to make amends but suffered betrayal. The following day, part of Mary's devotional included Psalm 22, and coming to verse 20, she read the words King David emphatically prayed,

Deliver me from the sword, my precious life from the power of

the dogs. (Psalms 22:20)

The movie's title depicted this one verse from the Bible. Now, the meaning of the movie rang with an augmented message of revelation: Betrayals are a plot of the enemy; they are the power of the dog.

Over the years, Mary has read this psalm many times, yet it was the first time her mind captured the expression "the power of the dog" with its resounding message. God, who breathed His own Spirit of life into us and rescued us from death, faced humanity's betrayal that sent Him to the cross. Similarly, in the story, the character who trusted his new friend faced a betrayal that led to his death. This is the power of the dog.

From the vantage point of this new revelation, Mary searched the entire Bible for further references. The words of Matthew 7:6 rang with an identical message.

Do not give dogs what is sacred; do not throw your pearls to

pigs. If you do, they may trample them under their feet, and

turn and tear you to pieces. (Matthew 7:6)

"Who are the dogs?" Mary asked God in prayer, and the Scripture once again outlined the answer.

Outside are the dogs, those who practice magic arts, the

sexually immoral, the murderers, the idolaters, and everyone

who loves and practices falsehood. (Revelation 22:15)

Further, the Prophet Isaiah explains how to recognize the power of the dogs in our lives.

They are dogs with mighty appetites; they never have enough.

They are shepherds who lack understanding; they all turn to

their own way, each seeks his own gain. (Isaiah 56:11)

For a few days, Mary lingered over this new understanding and prayed against the power of the dog in her own life and the life of her friends and family.

January 2022

By the first week of January, the excitement of Christmas and the adventures of the New Year have now all passed, permanently inscribed into the scrapbooks of old memories. Mary quickly directed her attention toward a newly developed task. She received an urgent request for biblical prayer counseling for a young woman, Laura, who was going through a family crisis. Laura was from Wisconsin and was visiting her mother, who lived in Burnet, Texas. Simultaneously, Laura sought counseling while staying with her mother. Through a string of extraordinary circumstances that unfolded over the holidays, Mary connected with Laura. It was beyond doubt that God had directed the paths of Laura and Mary to cross. It was God's divine appointment for Laura.

The night prior to the first meeting, Mary asked the Lord for direction. "The power of the dog," she heard the voice of the Lord. Was her mind lingering on the recent meditation on this topic, or was God directing her there? Mary was not entirely convinced. In the morning, before the first session, she inquired of the Lord for direction again. This time, the voice of the Lord was louder, "the power of the dog." Mary trusted God. She quickly put a one-page summary from the Scripture on "the power of the dog."

The first session began with Mary presenting Laura with the teachings on "the power of the dog" and the circumstances under which she was bringing this Scripture. She further pointed out that after watching the movie on Netflix with the same title, her devotional was on Psalm 22 the following day, where the expression "the power of the dogs" revealed a new profound meaning. And now, when she inquired of the Lord for direction, the same Scripture came up. Laura wept. Mary asked Laura to watch the Netflix movie for further discussions on the topic.

The following day, Laura appeared visually perplexed. She looked at Mary, bewildered, an expression radiating with amazement. Her entire body conveyed an internal steering of her spirit that aroused Mary's attention.

Through frequent, shallow breathing, Laura explained that she had committed to reading two psalms daily ten days earlier. Her devotion on the day after she watched the movie The Power of the Dog was Psalm 22. Coming to verse 20, Laura paused in disbelief because her experience mirrored Mary's experience. Both women locked eyes for a long moment, overwhelmed with the realization of the truth spoken. In the silence of that moment, they both heard God's voice loud and clear: "The Power of the Dog" was not only a movie; it was the root of Laura's problem.

The Lord God had created this very moment for Laura and Mary, where the revelation of Scripture and life experiences would bond in truth revealed. God caused their identical experience with Psalm 22 to amplify His message. God loved Laura, and He moved mountains to deliver the needed help. God entrusted the task to Mary, with whom He had a long history of a faith-driven relationship. This is one of the rare occasions when God used a Hollywood production to bring glory to His name.

After an intense week of counseling, Laura returned home to Wisconsin. Six months later, Mary received a text message from Laura, saying, "The power of the dog no longer has power over my family. Thank you."

Question: Have you experienced the "power of the dog" in your life? Were you the victim or the perpetrator?

_____

_____

_____

_____

_____

_____

_____

EHAD with GOD

REFLECTION—Week Seven

Reflection 1: Give Him 5—practicing God's presence (see description on pages 41 and 63 under "Deep calls to deep " section)

Reflection 2: Daily confession and repentance in prayer to Christ—our high priest; crucify the flesh, wash with the blood, fill with the Holy Spirit (page 13)

Reflection 3: The Story of Dan

The Story of Dan

When they asked for a volunteer, I didn't think twice and came forward. The heaviness bubbling from deep within has now surfaced, its full force threatening my very existence. I was good at putting a lid on it for many years, but not at that time. At that moment, the build-up was at the point of no return, amounting to an explosion. Stepping forward was a surrender to the unbearable pressure inside, with the hope of relieving it. To this day, I know that neither bravery nor pain moved me to step forward. God's divine providence propelled me to volunteer that day; I just agreed to submit to His guidance.

In all sincerity, I have never imagined that I would ever find myself as a volunteer in my Biblical Counseling class at the seminary I was attending. Two days of foundational teachings were followed by hands-on practice. As pastoral counselors in training, we had to start the healing with ourselves. Just like Lord Jesus, we were to become those wounded healers for the healing of many.

Twenty-two of us in the class have traveled hundreds of miles to attend this intensive training. We have never met previously; we have only become acquainted with each other through sharing about our ministries. The desire to learn the things of God was the single driving force for all of us to work as one.

The professor called two other students, who at the time served as a pastor and a worship leader in different congregations in different parts of the country. They were instructed to lay hands on me and to listen to the Holy Spirit for direction. The professor began with a short prayer. The sound of his first words opened a flood that swept over me. Just like with King David, in the days past, God's breakers and waves were crashing over me at that moment as well (Psalms 42:7). Tears began rolling down my face, and my shoulders hunched low, convulsing under the silent cries.

The professor's voice resounded, clear and steady, "Heavenly Father, we come before your throne of grace, bringing our friend for your divine healing. He is your earthen vessel (2 Corinthians 4:7). Restore him. Put together the broken pieces of his life. Cleanse him with the power of your blood spilled on the cross. Fill him with your Holy Spirit, sanctify him with your presence, and use him for honorable purposes. In Jesus' name, we pray, Amen!"

The pastor and the youth minister followed with short prayers, but their words bounced back, unable to reach my hearing. My sorrow had shrouded my senses with pain. My tears were now a torrent, matching the turmoil inside.

Silence followed. Then, the pastor's voice emerged, gaining strength with each word spoken, drawing my attention, "When the professor prayed of an earthy vessel to be restored, cleansed, sanctified, and used for honorable purposes, I had a vision of a young boy running up and down on a seashore picking up pottery pieces, trying to put them together... but one piece kept falling off. What does this mean?"

The youth minister also spoke, his voice sounding equally bewildered. "While the professor prayed, I saw hands putting together pottery pieces, and I also saw one piece missing. What is this, professor?"

My attention was aroused. The visions during prayer were about me. Silence forced itself into the classroom again, this time loaded with expectation.

And then, out of the far corner of the room, the voice of a young student rose steady and clear, "God forgave him, but he cannot forgive himself."

Everyone understood that the missing pottery piece was my inability to forgive myself. I didn't know that the disgust with myself over my past life choices had such grave consequences. My battle with guilt and self-condemnation, which was now made public for everyone to see, had just begun.

Ever since my teenage years, I got hooked on a bad crowd. Drugs, alcohol, and parties were my daily routines. The theft was the way to pay for my "extravaganza" lifestyle. I became addicted, and my addiction demanded constant fueling. I did many bad things: I robbed and destroyed property, I did violence, and I hurt people. The cops finally caught up with me and threw me in prison. For twelve long years, I was locked behind bars for good.

I reasoned that God, who is holy and righteous, cannot overlook my past offenses. With this set of mind, I drowned in guilt, suffocating the joy of my salvation. The message through the prayers took hold of that understanding and shattered it, now exposing my guilt as an offense. The only way forward was my response of contrition, confession, and repentance. The act of turning away from believing the lies of the Devil marked my way to freedom from guilt. Prophet Malachi had accurately described my new state of mind and heart.

> But for you who fear my name, the sun of righteousness shall
> rise, with healing in its wings. You shall go forth leaping like
> calves from the stall. (Malachi 4:2)

At that time, I was the "calf" leaping from my imprisonment to guilt into freedom. This is my most incredible healing story. I testify to the healing because it happened to me. The missing piece was found. It was my guilt. My healing put back together that missing piece and made my vessel whole. God is now using me for the honorable purpose of expanding His Kingdom on earth.

Task: Identify areas of your life that are plagued with guilt.

_____

_____

_____

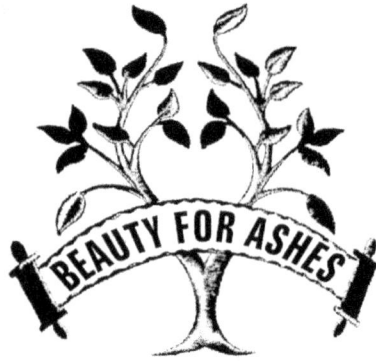

SESSION EIGHT

GENERATIONAL CURSES

The Law of Moses And Generational Curses

Generational blessings and curses are embedded in the Law of Moses, the Ten Commandments. The first commandment postulates:

> I am the LORD your God, who brought you out of the land of Egypt, out of the land of slavery. You shall have no other gods before me. You shall not make for yourself an idol in the form of anything in heaven above, or in the earth beneath, or in the water below. You shall not bow down to them or worship them; for I, the LORD your God, am a jealous God, punishing the children for the sin of the fathers to the third and fourth generation of those who hate me, but showing love to a thousand [generations] of those who love me and keep my commandments. (Exodus 20:2-6)

The Law of God comes with blessings (Deuteronomy 28:1-13) and curses (Deuteronomy 27:15-26; 28:15-68). In session three, we discussed in detail how the blessings and the curses result in life or death, respectively. The teaching in the Scripture is consistent—obedience to the Law brings blessings and life; disobedience to the Law puts a curse and brings death (spiritual) on the person committing the offense. Breaking any of the commandments is a grievous sin. The first commandment, especially, as Jesus emphasized, is the pillar on which the rest of the commandments are hinged (Matthew 22:36-40). It evokes a blessing or a curse (Exodus 20:6). The sin, if not confessed and repented, is passed on to the next generation via bloodline genealogy.

The prophet Zachariah is given a vision of a flying scroll, containing the curses. The Israelites have defiled the land with their abominable practices, and they had to bear the consequences.

> And he said to me, "This is the curse that is going out over the whole land; for according to what it says on one side, every thief will be banished, and according to what it says on the other, everyone who swears falsely will be banished.
>
> The Lord Almighty declares, 'I will send it out, and it will enter the house of the thief and the house of anyone who swears falsely by my name. It will remain in that house and destroy it completely, both its timbers and its stones.'" (Zachariah 5:1-4)

Six hundred years after the giving of the Law of Moses, the Prophet Jeremiah validated the truthfulness of the blessings and the curses over a person's life.

> This is what the LORD says: "Cursed is the one who trusts in man, who depends on flesh for his strength and whose heart turns away from the LORD. He will be like a bush in the wastelands; he will not see prosperity when it comes. He will dwell in the parched places of the desert, in a salt land where no one lives." (Jeremiah 17:5-6)

After another six hundred years, following the Prophet Jeremiah's warning, Jesus also confirmed the validity of this same teaching, saying,

Do not think that I have come to abolish the Law or the Prophets; I have not come to abolish them but to fulfill them. I tell you the truth, until heaven and earth disappear, not the smallest letter, not the least stroke of a pen, will by any means disappear from the Law until everything is accomplished. (Matthew 5:17-18)

According to Jesus, as long as the heaven and earth stand, so will the Law of God, and the blessings and curses associated with it. As of today, the new order of things, the new heaven and the new earth, are future events for us (Revelation 21:1); thus, making the Law valid in our lives.

The curse is a spiritual state that evokes spiritual death, and according to the Law, it is passed on to the next generation. God is three-in-one: God the Father, the Son, and God the Holy Spirit. Humans, made after God's likeness, are created after the same three-in-one pattern: Body, soul, and spirit. Just as the physical resemblance and character traits are passed on from generation to generation, the spiritual resemblance is passed on in the same manner (1 Corinthians 15:46-49). Thus, the children not only inherit the physical resemblance of their parents but also the spiritual state of blessings or curses they have accrued.

The Curse of the Law

The Apostle Paul says that Christ redeemed us from the curse associated with the Law that results in death (Galatians 3:13). Yet, Christ says that He didn't come to abolish the Law but to fulfill it; as long as the heaven and earth exist, the Law is still valid (Matthew 5:17-18). How do we reconcile both statements? Is there a controversy? Or is there a misunderstanding of spiritual matters? What is the spiritual mechanism through which the blessings and the curses manifest in the life of the believer?

There is no difference between the above two Scriptures. Jesus and Apostle Paul both refer to the new reality of a person born again in Christ.

Jesus didn't abolish the Law. He did not lower the standard for His followers either. Instead, He imputed in the believers His righteousness, thus enabling them to live according to His righteous decrees. Because of the imputed righteousness, the believers are capable of not breaking the Law, thus negating the power of death. The fulfillment of the Law in the life of the believers is manifested by their ability to meet the righteous requirements of the Law. There is no need to work for one's righteousness. Christ's righteousness has become an inherent part of believers' character. Therefore, no exertion in keeping with the Law is needed. Just through simple, child-like faith in Christ, God imputes in the believer His righteousness, the ability to live out the righteous requirements of the Law.

This is the spiritual mechanism through which Jesus canceled the spiritual curse. He is the One who enables the believer to live a righteous life. His presence in the believers' hearts changes the believers' character. Meeting the righteous requirements of the Law becomes the most natural way of life for a believer. This is a fulfillment of an ancient prophecy of which the believers are the beneficiaries.

> This is the covenant I will make with the people of Israel
> after that time," declares the Lord. "I will put my law in
> their minds and write it on their hearts. I will be their God,
> and they will be my people. (Jeremiah 31:33)
> I will give them an undivided heart and put a new spirit in
> them; I will remove from them their heart of stone and
> give them a heart of flesh. Then they will follow my decrees
> and be careful to keep my laws. (Ezekiel 11:19-20)
> I will give you a new heart and put a new spirit in you; I
> will remove from you your heart of stone and give you a
> heart of flesh. And I will put my Spirit in you and move you
> to follow my decrees and be careful to keep my laws.
> (Ezekiel 36:26,27)

The Law is like an instruction manual, guiding humanity in preserving spiritual life under the corrupt circumstances of the fallen world. Throughout the Scripture, God repeatedly warned the Israelites that idolatry results in death, triggering the curses of the Law, especially the curses associated with the first commandment.

> Say to them, 'As surely as I live,' declares the Sovereign LORD,
> 'I take no pleasure in the death of the wicked, but rather that
> they turn from their ways and live. Turn! Turn from your evil
> ways! Why will you die, O house of Israel?' (Ezekiel 33:11)

Living under the Law in Old Testament times must have been very dreadful. The Temple system was pedantically legalistic to meet the righteous requirements of the Law of God. Only through the Law does one become conscious of sin (Romans 5:20). The Law determines what is sinful and what is righteous. It sets eternal universal moral standards according to which spiritual and physical realms function.

> The sting of death is sin, and the power of sin is the law. (1
> Corinthians 15:56)

No matter how hard the Israelites worked to keep the Law, it was unattainable by any human means (Romans 3:10-12; Psalm 14:1-3; Psalms 53:1-3). It is still unattainable to this day unless the believers attain the righteousness of Christ, which enables them to meet the righteous requirements of the Law.

> Not having a righteousness of my own that comes from the
> law, but that which is through faith in Christ—the
> righteousness that comes from God and is by faith.
> (Philippians 3:9)

Jesus went to the cross on His free will and became the guilt offering needed for the redemption of humanity from the curse of the Law—death due to the consequences of sins. On the cross, He took the curse associated with the

Law of God—death—upon Himself. At that moment, all the sins of the world were put on Him. (1 John 2:2)

> God did [cancel the deadly power of the Law] by sending his own Son in the likeness of sinful man to be a sin offering. And so he condemned sin in sinful man, in order that the righteous requirements of the law might be fully met in us, who do not live according to the sinful nature but according to the Spirit. (Romans 8:3,4)
>
> God made him who had no sin to be sin for us, so that in him we might become the righteousness of God. (2 Corinthians 5:21)

Death through being "hanged on a tree" is the destiny of a lawbreaker. Despite being completely innocent, Jesus was counted among the lawbreakers because the iniquity of the entire humanity weighed on Him. From a human perspective, Jesus paid the penalties and suffered the punishment of death on the cross. It appeared that the enemy, the Devil, succeeded in killing the Son of God, thus thwarting his own ultimate demise. From heaven's perspective, however, the punishment of death was a spiritual transaction through which Jesus, God Himself, became the substitute offering for believers' death sentence. From that punishment of death sprang life, not only for Jesus upon His resurrection, but to all who would believe in Him; He granted life into eternity. Who is the loser, then? Jesus rose on the third day, alive and powerful, transformed from the helpless state of a sacrificial lamb on the cross to the Lion of Judah, the King of Kings, and the Lord of Lords in heaven. Death had no hold on Him (Acts 2:24). The tomb could not keep Him down. He defeated death for eternity, for all humanity.

> Where, O death, is your victory? Where, O death, is your sting? (1 Corinthians 15:55)

What happened to Jesus will happen to all who believe in Him. He was the firstborn from the dead (Colossians 1:18). Through Jesus, all who believe in Him also defeated death.

> Therefore, there is now no condemnation for those who are in Christ Jesus, because through Christ Jesus the law of the Spirit of life has set me free from the law of sin and death. (Romans 8:1)

Since believers become heirs with Christ (Romans 8:17), they are grafted onto His genealogy (Romans 11:11-31) and inherit the benefit of His victory over death. There is a condition to inherit this great blessing: Keep His commandments; specifically significant is obedience to the first commandment: To love the Lord your God with all your heart and with all your soul and with all your mind (Matthew 22:37-39). The righteous requirements of the Law of God never changed. Jesus made it clear that obedience to the first commandment not only shatters curses but brings the ultimate blessing of becoming EHAD with God:

> If anyone loves me, he will obey my teaching. My Father will love him, and we will come to him and make our home with him [become EHAD with him]. (John 14:24)

The eternal consequence of this victory has a new spiritual reality—Christ in you, the hope of glory (Colossians 1:27). What happens when a believer breaks the Law of God? The Holy Spirit convicts the believer of wrongdoing, producing godly sorrow that leads to life (2 Corinthians 7:10). There is a provision in the Law that stipulates,

> And when you and your children return to the LORD your God and obey him with all your heart and with all your soul according to everything I command you today, then the LORD your God will restore your fortunes and have compassion on you ... The LORD will again delight in you and make you prosperous, just as he delighted in your fathers, if you obey

the LORD your God and keep his commands and decrees that
are written in this Book of the Law and turn to the LORD your
God with all your heart and with all your soul. (Deuteronomy
30:2-10)

Indeed, when believers deviate from the narrow road that leads to eternal life (Matthew 7:14), Jesus leaves the ninety-nine and runs after them (Matthew 18:12). The moment you said "Yes" to Jesus, you were saved. Just as the Israelites entered into a covenant with the living God on Mount Sinai, you also entered into a covenantal relationship with the living God. God never abandoned Israel; God will never abandon you. The condition, though, of loving the Lord with all your heart and with all your soul remains in effect. Thus, the call to "work out your salvation with fear and trembling" (Philippians 2:12) is a reminder that the only required "work" from the believer is to love the Lord with all your heart and with all your soul and with all your mind (Matthew 22:37-39). Do not dwell in the past; once repented, God wipes it out.

Forget what is behind and strain toward what is ahead, press
on toward the goal to win the prize for which God has called
you heavenward in Christ Jesus. (Philippians 3:14)

Generational Curses and Familial Spirits

Sinful behavior feels "natural" to the person. For example, a spirit of pornography, homosexuality, transgenderism, addictions to drugs and alcohol, bouts of anger and rage would feel like an inborn tendency or character traits that are hard to change. From a spiritual perspective, these conditions indicate the presence of an unclean spirit. The only way to evict the unwanted spiritual occupier is penitence for committing the sinful offense. When the offense is generational, one must confess and repent of their own sin and confess and repent on behalf of the ancestors' sin, all the way down, genealogically, to the last known generation associated with the sin. In the book of Leviticus, God declares that He will forgive his people if "they confess their iniquity and the iniquity of their fathers."

> Those of you who are left will waste away in the lands of their enemies because of their sins; also because of their ancestors' sins they will waste away. But if they will confess their sins and the sins of their fathers—their treachery against me and their hostility toward me, which made me hostile toward them so that I sent them into the land of their enemies—then when their uncircumcised hearts are humbled, and they pay for their sin, I will remember my covenant with Jacob and my covenant with Isaac and my covenant with Abraham, and I will remember the land. (Leviticus 26:39-42)

However, if the sins are not confessed and forgiven, they are passed on to the next generation, along with the spirits attached to them. This is a spiritual transaction based on the unmovable principles of the Law. In the spiritual realm, the parents have the highest level of spiritual authority and responsibility over their children (Deuteronomy 6:4-6). Within the familial unit, parents become conduits of God's blessings or curses. Rebellious spiritual choices of the parents open doors for evil spiritual entities to establish themselves in their lives and, consequently, in the lives of their offspring. Since the spiritual entities have been allowed to take residence in parents' lives, that would automatically give them legal permission and access to the children. Thus, from generation to generation, the curse, associated with the sins of the forefathers, is passed onto the third and the fourth generation (Exodus 20:2-6) unless the sin is confessed and repented.

Consecutive generations suffer because of the sins of their forefathers. To be clear, it is not the sins of the fathers that are passed on to the children; the children are not considered guilty. It is, rather, the consequences of the sins of the fathers that afflict the children. This accounts for what today is known as a hereditary predisposition towards certain practices and behaviors. For example, alcoholism, drug addiction, promiscuity, sexual deviance, etc., are considered hereditary. The parents' practice of certain behaviors increases the likelihood of the consecutive generations exhibiting the same behavior.

This dynamic, undoubtedly, manifested in the life of Ben[13]. He was adopted as an infant into a Christian home. He was raised in multiple mission fields around the globe and accepted Christ at a very young age. At the age of 14, he met his biological father and encountered stunning similarities. The father was raped at the age of 6, and so was Ben. The father had a rebellious character, and so did Ben. The father was addicted to drugs and alcohol, and Ben was going down the same trajectory, using and selling drugs in high school. Even though the biological father had no physical presence in his life to influence Ben's behavior and choices, Ben nevertheless ended up on the same downward course as his biological father. The adoptive parents' drug-free and violence-free environment that Ben lived in was overridden by the curse in his bloodline. The familiar spirits associated with the sin of the father followed Ben. It is a spiritual Law.

This kind of behavioral genetics has been recognized and is even being considered as defense evidence in the court of law that might impact determinations of criminal responsibility and sentencing[14]. The understanding tends to remove the offenders' guilt since they are not responsible for the inborn genetics they had inherited, thus resulting in a lesser penalty.

From a biblical perspective, the observed behaviors are physical manifestations of spiritual reality. They constitute the spiritual heredity passed on along the bloodline. Within the family, an innocent child is exposed to spiritual entities that influence the parents' lives. The church sacrament of child baptism (Catholic and Orthodox Church) and child blessing and dedication (Evangelical Church) evoke a shield of protection over the child. Nevertheless, daily exposure to a sinful family environment makes the

---

[13] https://youtu.be/32N5Jc9GLtY?si=VGCHhcjVCBeYycDc

[14] Sabatello M, Appelbaum PS. Behavioral Genetics in Criminal and Civil Courts. Harv Rev Psychiatry. 2017 Nov/Dec;25(6):289-301.

defenseless child a vulnerable target against the spiritual forces of darkness and is more likely to succumb to their assault. The child internalizes his parents' behavior as "normal" and starts to embody it in his/her own actions. This spiritual condition is visually manifested when the child starts exhibiting the parents' symptomatic behavior. At this point, the sins of the parent have passed on to the child, who is now fully engaged in the same sinful practice, and as a consequence, just as the parent, the child is placed under the curse of the Law. If the child, as a believer, confesses the sin and turns away from the sinful practice, the child is legally cleared from the penalty of the offense. If the parents, however, never confessed and repented of their sins, their offense creates an outstanding spiritual debt that is transferred to the child, even though the child has been redeemed. The child is not considered sinful, but the child's life is affected by the ancestors' sins, as described above. This hypothetical spiritual situation may be a possible explanation for the question, "Why do bad things happen to good people?" The only scriptural way to cancel the curses associated with the Law is confession and repentance on behalf of the ancestors (Leviticus 26:39-42), especially ancestors who are deceased and can no longer do so.

Daniel (Daniel 9:16), Ezra (Ezra 9:6–7), and Nehemiah (Nehemiah 1:5; 9:2) practiced the virtue of confession and repentance for the sins of the forefathers. According to the instructions in Leviticus 26:39-42, one must: 1) repent for their own sins and then 2) repent for the sins of their ancestors. The Bible directs us to repent from the guilt of our ancestors because we have inherited the obligation to atone for their mistakes. The physical death of past generations does not cancel the spiritual trespass of the sins committed long ago. They, instead, extend to the next generation as outstanding spiritual debt.

Individual and Generational Judgment

There are two seemingly contradictory statements. On the one hand, Scripture tells us that each individual should bear the guilt for their own sins.

In those days people will no longer say: "The fathers have eaten sour grapes, and the children's teeth are set on edge." Instead, everyone will die for his own sin; whoever eats sour grapes—his teeth will be set on edge. (Jeremiah 31:29–30)

On the other hand, Scripture says that God visits the guilt of fathers upon their children.

You show steadfast love to thousands, but you repay the punishment for fathers' sins into the laps of their children after them. (Jeremiah 32:18a)

How do we reconcile these two different scriptures spoken by the Prophet Jeremiah? They are not different. They both refer to the same Law. These two references describe two different outcomes of the same spiritual reality that governs the Law of God. The spiritual roots are identical and must be dealt with similarly through confession, repentance, and forgiveness.

Individual Judgment

Fathers shall not be put to death for their children, nor children put to death for their fathers. Each is to die for his own sin. (Deuteronomy 24:16)

The Prophet Ezekiel, like the Prophet Jeremiah, brings the same message.

For every living soul belongs to me, the father and the son— both alike belong to me. The soul who sins is the one who will die. (Ezekiel 18:4)

First, even though the retribution for sin is passed to the next generation, that generation, if righteous, is guilt-free. Life may not go well with that generation due to the outstanding generational debt, but the generation is not condemned. If the children reject the sinful practice of their parents, they are set free from the enslaving power of that particular sin. The debt of their parents' offense, however, is still outstanding. It is canceled only when the sins of the fathers are confessed and atoned for by the children, in a manner which Daniel, Ezra, and Nehemiah did (described below).

Second, the biblical references above are spoken prophetically for a time when the curses associated with the Law would be broken when Christ would cancel their power of death and destruction. This is a well-known biblical pattern of weaving through now and then, between the current and the prophetic; it is an example of what Jesus often referred to, "Let the reader understand" (Matthew 24:15), or "Whoever has ears let them hear" (Matthew 13:9;13:43;23:35; Luke 8:8;14:35; Mark 4:9). Today, the children of God are free from the guilt of their own sins. They have severed the generational curse. It will not be passed on to their children. However, there might be an outstanding guilt inherited from their ancestors. The guilt, once identified, must be confessed and repented immediately. Only then will the genealogical account be cleared of any spiritual debt. Such is the mechanism and the function of God's Law.

Today, the Law concerning generational sins, in Leviticus 26, continues to be in effect. Because of the power of the Cross of Christ, however, the dreadful consequences to the next generation are negated. There is a condition, though: To negate the guilt of fathers' sins upon the children, the sins of the fathers must be confessed and repented by the consecutive generation.

Despite the different spiritual implications of being "under the Law" (Old Testament) or "under grace" (New Testament), the outcome of generational curses is the same. The same is also the biblical way to negate them by repenting, renouncing, and atoning for the sins committed. Humility before God ultimately cancels the power of sin over consecutive generations. Scripture attests to this truth:

> Like a fluttering sparrow or a darting swallow, an undeserved
> curse does not come to rest. (Proverbs 26:2)

Generational Judgment

As mentioned earlier, the Law of God comes with blessings and curses. These are conditions that come with the covenant between God and His people. To this day, the postulations of the Law of God continue to be valid (Exodus

20:5,6; Deuteronomy 5:9). Prophet Jeremiah lamented because he recognized the exile as a generational judgment.

> Our fathers sinned, and are no more; and we bear their
> punishment. (Lamentations 5:7)

The Old Testament abounds with examples of children falling under the judgment of their fathers: The generation of Noah (Genesis 7:21), Sodom and Gomorrah (Genesis 19:24,25), and Ahab (1 Kings 21:21,22). The people asked Jesus if the condition of an invalid man was associated with this Law. He responded,

> "Neither this man nor his parents sinned," said Jesus, "but
> this happened so that the works of God might be displayed in
> his life." (John 9:3)

Jesus did not negate the existence of generational curses; He clarified the purpose of that man's condition. Suffering for the sins of a previous generation was a common explanation for the misfortunes in life at that time. Similar to ancient times, today we must attain the knowledge of how generational sins lead to negative consequences for future generations. We also must cancel the power of these generational sins by seeking repentance and forgiveness from God for ourselves and our forefathers. The sins of the father continue to affect the consecutive generations ONLY if they are not confessed and atoned for.

Task: Examine your family tree. Do you notice a pattern of persistent health conditions or behaviors that have carried on from generation to generation? Examples include alcoholism, depression, anger, violence, promiscuity, laziness, addictions, adultery, fear, high anxiety, or sexual deviations. How have these behaviors affected your life? Create a list of the issues in your ancestral bloodline that may have influenced your life.

_____
_____
_____
_____
_____

The Sins of the Fathers

The Bible records numerous prayers of confession, offered for the sins committed by previous generations (Daniel 9:4–19; Ezra 9:6–7). During King Manasseh's reign, Judah's idolatry was so prevalent that even after the king publicly repented, the people didn't follow his example. Instead, they remained steeped in sin. Manasseh's father, Hezekiah, walked before God in truth and did what was good in God's sight (2 Kings 20:3). But Manasseh set Judah on a course that would lead to exile in Babylon. There were no more "good kings" in Judah after him. Manasseh not only worshiped false gods, setting up altars to idols in the Temple, but he committed the ultimate abomination when he sacrificed his own son. In the blunt judgment of 2 Kings 21:2, Manasseh "did evil in the eyes of the Lord."

Manasseh, however, repented! He turned back to God, changed his ways, and reinstated the worship of God (2 Chronicles 33:12-13). Yes, Manasseh received forgiveness. On a personal level, his repentance was sincere, which positioned him to become right with God. However, the decades-long legacy of leading the nation of Judah in apostasy was insufficient to stop his people's spiritual decline. The people didn't repent. The damage during the reign of King Manasseh was irreversible for that generation. Even though Manasseh destroyed the altars to idols and reinstated true worship in God's Temple, the people never entirely gave up their abominable religious practices (2 Chronicles 34:3). A decade later, God, through Prophet Jeremiah, repeatedly pleaded with Judah to return to Him by confessing and repenting of their sins and the sins of their fathers.

> Return faithless Israel, declares the LORD. Only acknowledge your guilt—you have rebelled against the LORD your God. (Jeremiah 3:11b-13)

The people from Jeremiah's time acknowledged their sins.

We have sinned against the LORD our God, both we and our fathers; from our youth till this day, we have not obeyed the LORD our God. (Jeremiah 3:25b)

The acknowledgment of wrongdoing doesn't cancel the sin of committing it. Only confession and sincere repentance cancel the sin. Unfortunately, no one repented of their wickedness (Jeremiah 8:6), and Judah went into exile.

Seventy years into the exile, Prophet Daniel reads Jeremiah's writings and learns that the punishment for the rebellion would last seventy years.

"'This whole country will become a desolate wasteland, and these nations will serve the king of Babylon seventy years. But when the seventy years are fulfilled, I will punish the king of Babylon and his nation, the land of the Babylonians, for their guilt,' declares the LORD, 'and will make it desolate forever.' " (Jeremiah 25:11-12)

Prophet Daniel realizes that the seventy years of desolation are about to be completed, thus fulfilling the prophecy. He then applied the directives of Leviticus 26 and proceeded with confession and repentance on behalf of his people, Israel.

So I turned to the LORD God and pleaded with him in prayer, petition, fasting, sackcloth, and ashes. I prayed to the LORD my God and confessed: O LORD, the great and awesome God, who keeps his covenant of love with all who love him and obey his commands, we have sinned and done wrong. We have been wicked and have rebelled; we have turned away from your commands and laws. (Daniel 9:3-5)

These are the steps recorded in Daniel's prayer.

1) Penitent heart: Daniel pleaded with God in prayer and petition, in fasting, in sackcloth and ashes (Daniel 9:3).

2) Confession and repentance of personal sins: Daniel acknowledged and repented of his sins (Daniel 9:5).

3) Confession and repentance for the sins of the forefathers: Daniel prayed to the Lord, confessing the sins of his forefathers (Daniel 9:3-4).

4) Seeking and accepting God's forgiveness: Daniel pleaded for mercy (Daniel 39:15-18, 19).

The Scripture recorded that the Lord God heard Daniel's prayers and decreed the return of the Jews to their land. Similarly, Prophet Ezra prayed,

> O my God, I am too ashamed and disgraced to lift up my face
> to you, my God, because our sins are higher than our heads,
> and our guilt has reached to the heavens. From the days of our
> forefathers until now, our guilt has been great. Because of our
> sins, we and our kings and our priests have been subjected to
> the sword and captivity, to pillage and humiliation at the hand
> of foreign kings, as it is today. (Ezra 9:6–7)

God heard Ezra's prayers and enabled the Israelites to continue rebuilding the Temple of God.

Canceling Generational Sins

How do we practically apply the spiritual laws of confession and repentance in our lives? God heard the prophets' prayers and accepted them. He is equally moved by our entreaty and decrees changes. Today, believers' prayers can also actuate matters in the spiritual world because the Spirit has been poured on all flesh (Joel 2:28; Isaiah 32:15; Ezekiel 39:29; Zechariah 12:10; John 7:39). Through the victory of Christ on the cross, we are now judicially positioned, in prayer, to evoke changes in the spiritual and natural realms.

Just as the act of confession and repentance places an individual in right standing with God, so does the act of confession and repentance for the sins of the ancestors. Confession and repentance are spiritual tools that negate the destructive forces perpetuated from one generation to another in a vicious cycle of sin and death.

Spiritual Power and Spiritual Authority

Upon salvation, **power** is apportioned to each believer through the indwelling of the Holy Spirit. **Authority** is the legal right to exercise this power within our spiritual jurisdictions. The overarching spiritual jurisdiction on earth is Christ. The Church of God is under Christ and is in charge of caring for God's people. The Church, with its priestly office, forms the horizontal structures. It constitutes a powerful overarching jurisdiction for the protection of God's faithful believers. In their own terms, the believers also represent separate jurisdictions as apportioned within their own families. As the priests and pastors exercise their authority over their congregations and parishes, so can the families exercise their power and authority within their own familial jurisdictions. These sub-levels of jurisdiction within the Church form the vertical structures of power and authority. Christ is the head of the Church (Colossians 1:18). Ministers, pastors, priests, and elders are subject to Christ, functioning as His ambassadors. Families that are part of a church or parish form their jurisdiction. The jurisdiction of Christ, our Lord, God, and Savior, has an all-encompassing power over all structures and authorities. The believers remain protected and safe as long as they stay under these spiritual jurisdictions.

God assigned extraordinary spiritual jurisdictions within the family. Ephesians 5:21-33 stipulates the relational dynamics within the marriage. The husband himself is under the authority of Christ. The family is an eminent part of the vertical structures within the Church of Christ that ensure protection and safety.

> Wives, submit to your husbands as to the Lord. For the husband is the head of the wife as Christ is the head of the church, his body, of which he is the Savior. Now, as the church submits to Christ, so also wives should submit to their husbands in everything. (Ephesians 5:22-24)

These are God's appointed authority structures within the family and His Church. As long as family members operate within these structures, they are protected. If they venture outside these structures or altogether reject them, they no longer have God's full protection because they have placed themselves in the enemy's territory. Widows and single mothers are directly positioned under the office of the church/parish and ultimately under Christ's protection and authority. The responsibility to care for the widows and the orphans falls on the Church (Deuteronomy 24:17; Psalms 68:4-6; Proverbs 15:25; 1 Timothy 5:3-16; James 1:27).

Despite the levels of jurisdictional authority, every believer still has direct access to God (Hebrews 4:14-16; 5:6; 7:26-28; 9:11-12). Believers are endowed with power and authority within their familial boundaries; they constitute a divinely ordained spiritual jurisdiction. Every believer also has unique jurisdiction over their own body and the right to effect changes in their spiritual life. This is the "my home—my castle; my body—my life; my soul—my spirit" doctrine upon which every individual may exercise the right of free will and self-determination. Joshua exercised this authority, declaring:

> But as for me and my household, we will serve the LORD.
> (Joshua 24:15b)

Job also made a similar commitment,

> I made a covenant with my eyes not to look lustfully at a girl.
> (Job 31:1)

Jesus exemplified this marvelous authority, and every believer must model after Him. Commanding spiritual entities within one's personal jurisdiction is a power in believers' hands to counteract the schemes of the enemy. Just like Jesus, we must sternly employ the command:

> Get behind me, Satan! (Matthew 16:23)

Every child of God has the power and authority to command evil forces from the spiritual realm that affect their physical and spiritual life. You must put your foot down and say to the spiritual entities that are harassing your life,

"Get behind me, Satan!" The spiritual law governing persons' free will postulates that the spiritual entities must obey. They must vacate the "house" and move away to "arid places" (Matthew 12:43). They must stop harassing and oppressing the believer. This is your God-given, Christ-apportioned spiritual jurisdiction. You have full authority over your life. You are either with Christ or against Him; you either gather with Him or scatter (Matthew 12:30). The choice is yours.

Individuals who have experienced trauma due to physical or sexual abuse within their families are very vulnerable to evil influence. The stronghold of sin over the family must be destroyed, and the curse associated with the sin must be atoned. This stronghold can only be demolished through the spiritual act of confession and repentance for the sins of the fathers/mothers, as Leviticus 26 instructs.

The practice of sin within the family removes the cover of the God-given spiritual jurisdictional protections and places the individual/family under the jurisdiction of the enemy. For example, if the husband engages in sin, he no longer provides protection over his wife and children. They become vulnerable to the influence of the evil forces. Familial sins serve as a "foothold" for the enemy to do destruction; they give the enemy legal permission to enter and propagate evil (Ephesians 4:27). The only way to reverse this course of destruction and close the "access" door is to confess personal sins along with parents' sins, down to the known generations.

Children and Familial Jurisdiction

The children within the family are covered under the jurisdiction of the familial power and authority. This gives the right to parents to pray over their child/children, and because their prayers are spoken under the rightful jurisdiction within the family structure, they are effective in the spiritual realm. Below is an example of a parent's prayer over their children.

Parents' Prayer

Instruction: Place your hands over your child's head as you recite this prayer. Omit reading the biblical verse citations within the text—they are only for reference, confirming the words being prayed as trustworthy.

We, the parents of _____, stand united in the name of Jesus Christ, our Lord, God, and Savior, and by His power and authority vested in us, we claim the life of our child/children for the Kingdom of God. We pray life over you _____. We pray for the peace of Jesus in you. We pray for life in fullness for you (John 10:10). May your name be inscribed in the Book of Life (John 3:3; Revelation 20:15). May Jesus guide you on a path of righteousness. May His light be a light unto your feet (Psalms 119:105). May He give you the courage to choose what is right. May He give His angels charge over you (Psalms 91:11). May the Lord hear your prayers, answer them quickly, and grant your heart's desires (Psalms 20:19-22). May the Lord be near you and dispatch angels to your help (Psalms 91:11). May He protect you from the power of the dogs (Psalms 22); may lies and deception never seduce you.

May you learn to recognize the voice of the Lord amid the clutter of life (John 10:1-10). May the Law of God be inscribed on your heart and mind (Jeremiah 31:33, Hebrews 8:10b, 2 Corinthians 3:3). May the beauty of the Lord be upon you. May you grow to be a mighty oak of righteousness for the display of His splendor (Isaiah 61:3). May His righteousness be your righteousness, His holiness be your holiness, His joy be your joy, and His peace be your peace. May you spiritually grow in Christ from glory to glory (2 Corinthians 3:18). May your life be long and happy. May the spirit of poverty never come near your door. May you discern the Lord's plans, and may He give you the courage to stay on the path of pursuing them. May all your plans prosper (Jeremiah 29:11). God be with you for an abundant life!

For a boy: We claim the blessing of our spiritual ancestors for your life. May you inherit the blessings of Abraham, Isaac, Jacob, Moses, King David, the Prophet Daniel, the Apostles Paul, Peter, John, and the countless saints who walked with God in complete integrity. May the Lord assign you a likewise place of honor at His table (Luke 14:7-11). May the Spirit of the living God fall fresh on you (Ezekiel 36:27). May you serve Him in complete integrity of heart and mind. May He grant you the gifts of the Spirit according to your spiritual calling, as you serve before Him (Galatians 5:22-24). May you be a pillar of strength to guide many. May you always speak truthfully, and your words always be held in high esteem. May the Lord impart in you a Spirit of deep inquiry for His Word. May He reveal His deep mysteries to you. May He call you "friend" and speak with you face to face (John 15:15-17; Exodus 33:11). May the Lord make you the head, not the tail (Deuteronomy 28:13). May you never fall on your face. May your enemies flee from you in panic (Psalms 91). May the Lord provide a godly wife for you, a heavenly match for life. May your quiver be full (Psalms 127:3–5); may you be a father of many.

For a girl: We claim the blessings of our spiritual ancestors for your life. May you be like Sarah, Rebekah, Rachel, Leah, and Mary, the mother of Jesus, Mary Magdalene, and the countless other saints who walked with God in complete integrity. May the Lord assign you a likewise place of honor at His table (Luke 14:7-11). May the Spirit of the living God fall fresh on you (Ezekiel 36:27). May you be treasured more than rubies (Proverbs 31:10); may your beauty attest to the beauty of God, a display of his splendor (Isaiah 61:3). Walk before the Lord, your God, in complete integrity of heart and mind. May rivers of living waters flow out from you for the blessings of many (John 7:38). May deception be far from you (Psalms 22:19-22). May the eyes of the Lord scout the earth for a husband, a heavenly match for life. May you become a mother of many. May you manage your home with God's wisdom from above (Proverbs 24:3-4). May your children rise and call you blessed, and your husband praise you too (Proverbs 31:28). May the Lord bless the labor of your hands (Deuteronomy 28:12; Psalms 128:2-4).

Protection from evil

We command the forces of darkness to stay away from you. We pray for a hedge of protection over you (Job 1:8–11). Lord Jesus, we pray that you send angels to guard _____ continually (Psalms 91:11; Hebrews 1:14). Thwart any plans of the enemy directed towards _____ (Isaiah 54:15). Extinguish any fiery darts shot at _____ (Ephesians 6:10-18).

We break any curse spoken over _____ and nullify them (Galatians 3:13). We confess the sins of the forefathers and ask forgiveness for the offense (Leviticus 26). We break any curses coming from the mother's or father's generational lines and declare them invalid. We claim the blood of Christ over the generational lines and declare them cleansed. We place the helmet of salvation over _____'s head to protect him/her from worldly philosophies and teachings (Ephesians 6). We cut the access of evil to your life and command any entity not part of the Kingdom of God to flee from your presence. In Jesus' mighty name, see sealed these prayers with His blood and bless them with the covenant of His love.

Triple Priestly Blessings

May the LORD bless you and keep you. The LORD shine His face upon you and be gracious to you. The LORD turn His face toward you and give you peace [shalom] (Numbers 6:22).

We ask all this in the most precious name of Jesus. Amen!

EHAD with GOD

REFLECTION—Week Eight

Reflection 1: Give Him 5—practicing God's presence (see description on pages 41 and 63 under "Deep calls to deep" section)

Reflection 2: Daily confession and repentance in prayer to Christ—our high priest; crucify the flesh, wash with the blood, fill with the Holy Spirit (page 13)

Reflection 3: Confessing the Sins of My Forefathers

Reflection 4: Object Permanence—The Blind Side of Me

Reflection 5: The Story of Angela—One God, One Spirit

Confessing the Sins of My Ancestors

Task: Confession and repentance of personal sins and the sins of the forefathers are the biblical pathways for healing from trauma; they negate the destructive power of generational curses. Write your own prayer to reflect the afflictions within your own family.

_____

_____

_____

_____

_____

_____

_____

_____

_____

_____

_____

_____

Prayer

I speak these words in the presence of my Lord Jesus Christ. I call upon His holy name and ask Him, "Jesus, grant me the authority to command the demonic forces, familial spirits, and cancel the generational curses incurred on me through the bloodlines of my ancestors."

I confess Jesus as the Son of God who came in the flesh. He died for my sins, and His holy blood has made me clean. Jesus, I confess my sins and ask forgiveness for my trespasses. Please absolve me of my guilt. May Your power and authority flow through me right now. Give me the grace to overcome all things and confront the demons and the familial spirits trying to destroy me.

In the name of Jesus, I confess the sins of my ancestors and ask eternal forgiveness. May my confession and repentance of their iniquity block the demonic forces coming against me through the bloodline of my mother and father. I declare I am not responsible for their sins. I reject all agreements they have made with any demonic powers. On behalf of my ancestors, I confess any demonic contracts, vows, promises, obligations, assignments, or witchcraft and ask forgiveness for practicing them. I confess and ask forgiveness for their sins of manipulation, addiction, suicide, lust, perversion, hate, fear, anger, murder, divination, and the occult. I command the demons associated with these sins to lose their hold on me and my bloodlines now and forever. I pray the blood of Jesus over my bloodlines and declare them cleansed. I have no outstanding ancestral spiritual debt.

In the power and the authority vested in me by my Lord Jesus Christ, I now cancel all generational curses proceeding from the bloodlines of my mother and father. I say to the demonic entities that are attached to my bloodlines, "I cut your access to my life. Your work of darkness and power over me is canceled and nullified. You have no legal right over my life. You are evicted, be gone. Demons and familial spirits, you are not allowed to return. You are not permitted to send reinforcements or to attack any family member or loved ones. In the name of Jesus, be gone." Amen!

Object Permanence—The Blind Side of Me

Modern psychology defines the principle of "object permanence" as an intrinsic part of human development. It postulates that an object still exists even though not visible. This is why a child cries in distress when a caregiver leaves the room. Adults play "peek-a-boo" with young children, enforcing the notion of permanence. Object permanence is one of the major milestones of early childhood physical and emotional development. If one does not acquire an understanding of permanence at a very young age, problems with trust may be evidenced later in life.

Many believers, born again by the Spirit of God, have yet to achieve this critical spiritual milestone in their spiritual development. Out of their sorrowful experience, they have derived a wrong conclusion: If I cannot see God active in my healing, it means God's healing presence does not exist. Have you passed this spiritual milestone yet? Or, have you fallen into spiritual stagnation, readily accepting God's lack of involvement in your situation of pain and suffering rather than His immediate response to the healing?

Faith in Jesus is "blind." We don't believe because we have seen or our hands have touched (1 John 1:1); we believe because the Spirit of the Living God testifies with our spirit that we are children of the Most High (Romans 8:16). When we negate God's sovereignty in our healing, we are left to tend to ourselves. Then, we become just like the people in the Prophet Jeremiah's days, who dug their own cisterns, broken cisterns that cannot hold water.

> My people have committed two sins: They have forsaken me,
> the spring of living water, and have dug their own cisterns,
> broken cisterns that cannot hold water. (Jeremiah 2:13)

Question: Are you digging your own cisterns? Have you forsaken the Spring of Living Water? Reflect on your understanding.

_____

_____

_____

_____

The Story of Angela—One God, One Spirit

Angela took a deep breath as silence invaded the space on both sides of the phone line. Her mind instantaneously reached out to God for guidance. What should her response be? The request seemed impossible. Would God honor such a request and grant a response? The Law of God is clear, "Do not put the LORD your God to the test" (Deuteronomy 6:16-25). Fear gripped her heart as this request resembled such a test.

"Please pray for me," Julia has asked, "The Lord gave me a vision as I prayed for guidance. Pray and ask the Lord to confirm His message through you. Tell me what the vision was and how to interpret it."

Throughout the years, Angela has received many prayer requests, but nothing compared to this one. "I will inquire on your behalf before the Lord." Angela agreed. Years ago, Angela had made a covenant with her lips to never speak out of her own imagination. If the Lord speaks, she would boldly proclaim the message, even from the rooftops, if needed. But, if the Lord would remain silent, so would she.

Very early the following day, Angela entered her routine prayer time with the Lord with a dreadful heart. She worshipped God as she approached His presence. Heavenly sweetness melted the fears away. In reverent humility, Angela began making requests on behalf of her friend.

"Jesus, I come on behalf of my friend, Julia. She is seeking confirmation of your message to her. I dare not overstep Your sacred spiritual boundary and my allotted jurisdiction under the office of Your servant. I ask forgiveness if this request appears to You as a test and grieves your Holy Spirit. I know my simple place in the eternal spiritual hierarchy, and I empty myself of any pride or wrong, self-seeking motives. My Lord and King, may I, just like Esther, be granted mercy as I enter Your presence and make my request."

"Lord Jesus, there is a biblical precedent of a similar request in the story of the Prophet Daniel (Daniel 2). King Nebuchadnezzar had dreams that troubled his mind. He summoned his magicians, enchanters, sorcerers, and astrologers to tell him what he had dreamed and interpret it. None of them could do it. When, in his anger, the king ordered all of them to be killed, Daniel stepped up and asked for more time to solve the mystery. In prayer and fasting, Daniel went before you, and you revealed to him Nebuchadnezzar's dream and its interpretation. I know that the same Spirit that revealed the mystery to Daniel now lives in me. If it pleases You, Jesus, help my friend and confirm the message You gave her by revealing it to me." Angela pleaded with the Lord, and He answered.

Irrelevant to time and space, a moving picture began unfolding in her mind's eyes. Two hands were gently scrubbing the feet of a very young woman who was enjoying the experience, soaking in a deep bathtub. The removal of very rough surfaces from the feet revealed glowing skin. In the same fashion, the hands moved on, washing and scrubbing the entire body. The scene resembled an ancient setting, mysteriously engulfed in a semi-revealing ambient light. There was the notion of multiple servants attending to this cleansing ritual, each with a specifically assigned role and function. At once, the point of view changed, and Angela watched from behind as the young woman rose graciously from the bathtub, her beauty emanating perfection of forms and purity. The sight took Angela's breath away. Long, dark hair richly flowed over the beautiful pale olive frame. The physical beauty, though exceptional by itself, was not the reason for Angela's astonishment. The remarkable state of the young woman's purity evoked her admiration. It was a cleanliness of heavenly order, radiating divine holiness. She was spotless in mind and body, soul and spirit. "The beauty of Cleopatra," Angela whispered. The short vision faded away, but its impression lingered in Angela's mind.

The following two days, Angela pondered the experience as she faithfully remained in prayer. On the third day, Angela called Julie back and told her about the vision. After a short pause, Julie quietly said, "It is not Cleopatra. It is Esther." Before becoming queen for King Xerxes, Esther had to undergo twelve months of beauty treatments—six months with oil of myrrh and six with perfumes and cosmetics (Esther 2:12). Similarly, Julie had to commit to a period of scrubbing and washing, replacing the old flesh with the newness of the Spirit of God, preparing herself for special service in the heavenly courts of the King of Kings, Lord Jesus. Angela wept, reverently giving glory and honor to the God of heaven, the Revealer of mysteries.

Esther had to undergo one year of specially designed cleansing rituals fitting for the king's future queen. The believer, through the Holy Spirit, can accelerate this process significantly. *EHAD with GOD* was designed with that purpose—to present you to the King, Lord Jesus, pure, spotless, and wrinkle-free. The journey on the narrow road is the journey of washing and cleansing, purifying and refining. This is the process of sanctification described in this methodology. Confession, repentance, and forgiveness are the scrubbing means through which the believer sheds the old flesh, being transformed into the likeness of the King Jesus Himself.

Task: Rate your purity level (sanctification) before and after committing to the *EHAD with GOD* methodology, 1 being the lowest and 10 the highest.

Before

1	2	3	4	5	6	7	8	9	10
○	○	○	○	○	○	○	○	○	○

After

1	2	3	4	5	6	7	8	9	10
○	○	○	○	○	○	○	○	○	○

Task: Discuss the results of your reflection.

_____

_____

_____

_____

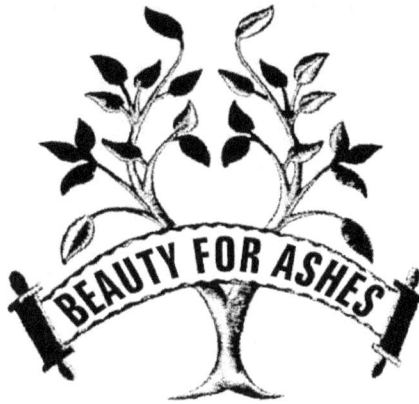

SESSION NINE

GLORIFICATION

Raham Agape Love

The corruption of the world has corrupted the meaning of love. The postmodern culture of this current age has blurred the boundaries between love and sex, proclaiming self-liberation from both. The bolder the declaration of this new love, the more overt the rebellion against the eternally established divine social norms. This new paradigm is displayed everywhere, from movies and covers of magazines to woke kindergarten children's books. Love has been taken down from the pedestal of sacred reverence, degraded to just "feel good," and promptly discarded when the feelings wear off. This new love has become the shallow understanding of good times of sensual passions over the lifetime commitment to loyal passions. There is an ugly irony in this postmodern progress: The liberation from love has resulted in love's annihilation. The consequence is a rejection of God's divine love, replacing it with the idol of self-indulgence in sensual love.

And yet, there is a deep longing for pure, honest, and loyal love. Filling with anything else deepens the yearning and widens the want. Love is an imminent part of the divinely designed human nature. This kind of love is stamped with God's royal approval. It is crowned with God's beauty. It is a blessed gift to humanity with which God made our lives abundant (John 10:10). The search for this love is an ever-eluding endeavor, often ending up overwhelmingly in disappointment rather than satisfaction. Does this true love exist? Yes, some have loved. Yes, we have heard their stories. And now, this is a prayer over your life of love: May your life story be a love story that you pass to the next generation of believers to inspire them to pursue their own love story, which they, in their turn, will pass on to the next generation of believers. Thus, from generation to generation, the truth of this divinely imparted love may never be forgotten. The name of this love is RAHAM (רחמ) in Hebrew/Aramaic and AGAPE (ἀγάπη) in Greek.

The English language doesn't distinguish between different degrees of love. In the same breath, we say "I love God" as well as "I love peanuts" or "I love my dad" or "I love my dog," "I love this song/painting/etc," for example. The degree of emotion invested in each of the above statements is different. The word "love" in English, for each statement, however, doesn't convey the intensity or the specificity of the emotions involved. Not so in the Hebrew, Aramaic, and the Greek languages.

In the ancient Greek language, the Scripture refers to three kinds of love: agape (ἀγάπη), phileo (φιλέω), and eros (ἔρως). Agape is the divinely imparted ability to love unconditionally; phileo is brotherly love, and eros is embedded in the command to procreate, which comes with the divine gift of sexual intimacy and pleasure.

Chaim Bentorah, a Biblical Hebrew scholar and bestselling author, explores the deeper meaning of love as written in the original languages of

Hebrew and Aramaic.[15] There are two Hebrew/Aramaic words which in the English Bible are translated as "love": RAHAM (רחם)(same in Hebrew and Aramaic) and AHAV (אהב) (Hebrew), HAV (Aramaic). RAHAM (רחם) depicts the divine love God has for humanity, for each human being. RAHAM (רחם) is a love in its purest form; a love that has not offended or wounded the heart of the Father. HAV (Aramaic) or AHAV (אהב) (Hebrew) is the rendering of brotherly love. The corresponding words of RAHAM and AHAV/HAV in the Greek language are AGAPE (ἀγάπη) and PHILEO (φιλέω).

RAHAM (רחם) is used 47 times in the Bible, with only three times found in the first five books of the Bible, the Torah (Exodus 33:19, Deuteronomy 13:17b, Deuteronomy 30:3). These three references are all translated in English as "mercy." RAHAM is God's intense love for us, a love that includes tender mercy, forgiveness, and compassion. These are the attributes of "agape love" that the Apostle Paul describes in 1 Corinthians 13.

There is only one time in the Bible when RAHAM describes a human's love for God, that of King David's love for God in Psalm 18:1. Even then, King David uses the word RAHAM (רחם) in its simple verbal Qal form, not daring to use it in its intensive form as applied to God's love for us (Aramaic as Pael, and Piel in Hebrew)[16]. King David, the man after God's own heart, could not love with the intensity of God's RAHAM (רחם) love. The English language falls short in making the distinction. This "raham" level of love is only possible with God and through God. King David found himself unable to reciprocate God's pure RAHAM (רחם) love for him.

The Word RAHAM (רחם) also means "womb" and is an expression of a mother's love for the fetus. By choosing RAHAM (רחם) over AHAV (אהב), King

---

[15] Chaim Bentorah (2020). Racham: The Love That is Beyond Love. True Potential, Inc, South Carolina

[16] Ibid., p. 63

David declares that his love for God arises from within him. As a mother is inseparable from the fetus, so is King David's bond to God an inherent part of his existence. It is a deep emotional tie between his spirit and God's Spirit that transcends into eternity. In Psalm 18:1, by his choice of RAHAM (רחמ), King David makes a public declaration that he belongs to God, "ארחמך יהוה" (Arahameha YHWH), "I love you God."

How do we measure up to God's RAHAM love for us? Can we reciprocate and love God with the same intensity and purity with which He loves us? Every committed believer wants to love the Lord with all their heart, soul, and strength. This is, after all, the first commandment. It is our desire, but is it a reality in our lives? How do we, then, attain this intense RAHAM AGAPE love?

Question: Are you able, just as King David, to declare your RAHAM love to God by saying, "ארחמך יהוה" - Arahameha YHWH - I love you, God. This level of pure love is only possible when one becomes EHAD with God. Are you there yet?

_____
_____
_____
_____
_____
_____
_____
_____
_____
_____
_____
_____
_____
_____

Raham Agape Love Reciprocated

After His resurrection, Jesus appeared to the disciples at the Sea of Galilee's shore, asking Peter three times if Peter loved Him.

> When they had finished eating, Jesus said to Simon Peter, "Simon son of John, do you truly love me more than these?" "Yes, Lord," he said, "you know that I love you." Jesus said, "Feed my lambs." Again, Jesus said, "Simon, son of John, do you truly love me?" He answered, "Yes, Lord, you know that I love you." Jesus said, "Take care of my sheep." The third time he said to him, "Simon, son of John, do you love me?" Peter was hurt because Jesus asked him the third time, "Do you love me?" He said, "Lord, you know all things; you know that I love you." Jesus said, "Feed my sheep." (John 21: 15-17)

The first two questions, "Do you love me?" in Greek, Jesus used the word "agape," which refers to God's divine, unconditional love. Both times, Peter responded, "I love you," using the Greek word "phileo," which refers to a brotherly kind of love. When asked the third time, Jesus Himself used the word "phileo" and received a "phileo" response from Peter again. At that time, Peter's love for Jesus was truly brotherly (phileo). Peter was honest. He had just failed to display agape love for Jesus, denying him three times. Peter recognized that his "phileo" love for Jesus could not match Jesus' "agape" love for Peter. Peter could not love on an agape level.

The above dialogue was originally spoken in the Aramaic language, with corresponding words being "raham" for "agape" and "hav" for phileo. Jesus didn't scold Peter for not being able to love him with agape love. He knew that this would soon change. In retrospect, Peter understood, too, because, after his transformation, his letters breathed agape love for his brothers and sisters in Christ. He also urged all to exhibit agape love (1 Peter 1:22,23; 2:17; 4:8; 5:4; 2 Peter 1:7). What caused the change in Apostle Peter's preference of word choice? How did Apostle Peter move from "phileo" love to "agape love?" It is simple. Both occasions are separated by a watershed moment, an event that divided the human understanding of God and His Kingdom before and after—the giving of the Holy Spirit on the Day of Pentecost.

The disciples learned and practiced under Jesus for three years, yet their knowledge was not internalized. Jesus granted them occasional power and authority to minister the gospel to others (Luke 10:1-18), but they had not yet experienced the indwelling power of the Holy Spirit. Before His resurrection, Jesus promised to send the Advocate, the Holy Spirit, who would remind them of His teachings and instruct them in the deep things of God (John 14:25-26). Only upon the Holy Spirit's indwelling power could the Apostle Peter reciprocate with agape love for the agape love of Jesus. Just like King David, Apostle Peter could now say, "I love [raham] you, Lord" (Psalms 18:1)

Attaining agape love is the prerequisite for EHAD with God. God is love—God is agape (1 John 4:8). We are made after His own image and likeness. Agape love was part of God's initial divine design. Humanity lost the capacity to agape love in the Garden of Eden, but Jesus restored it on the cross. Through sanctification, we attain agape love anew; we regain the capacity to reciprocate with agape love. Because God is agape, we become agape also. Mutual agape love is the solidifying component of being EHAD with God.

The presence of agape love attests to a transformative, enduring faith in the believer's life (1 Corinthians 13:5). It is a new, higher level of spiritual maturity. Jesus repeatedly equated agape love with obedience to His commandments.

> Whoever has my commands and keeps them is the one who
> loves [agape] me. (John 14:21)

Obedience to the Law of God attests to the impartation of Christ's righteousness through which He enables us to obey His commandments. Loving Jesus with agape love is a display of a higher level of spiritual growth at which the Law of God is inscribed in the heart (Romans 2:12-16; 1 Corinthians 3:3; Ezekiel 11:19). At this level of maturity, the Law becomes a permanent character trait. The command to "Love the Lord with all your heart, all your soul, with all your strength" (Matthew 22:37-39) is not a fearful obligation anymore; to love God on an agape level becomes the greatest delight in life.

In becoming EHAD with Jesus, which is sanctification and transformation in His image, you have so internalized God's Law that it has become your nature. You have arrived at a new mountain top of height, a new exhilarating flight of the human spirit, at which you can truly experience heaven on earth. At this point, Scripture refers to the believers who have achieved this spiritual maturity as becoming the Bride of Christ, who has made herself ready for her groom.

> Let us rejoice and be glad and give him glory! For the wedding
> of the Lamb has come, and his bride has made herself ready.
> Fine linen, bright and clean, was given her to wear.
> (Revelation 19:7-8)

Apostle Paul describes the required spiritual condition of becoming the Bride of Christ.

> To present her to himself as a radiant church, without stain or
> wrinkle or any other blemish, but holy and blameless.
> (Ephesians 5:27)

Holiness and purity are signs of spiritual maturity in becoming EHAD with Christ. Without holiness, no one will see the Lord (Hebrews 12:14). The grand finale in the Scripture reaches a crescendo with the image of the betrothal unity of Christ and His Bride, the Church, as we truly become EHAD.

> The Spirit and the Bride say, "Come." And let him who hears
> say, "Come." Whoever is thirsty, let him come; and whoever
> wishes, let him take the free gift of the water of life.
> (Revelation 22:17)

Even more, this elevated state of spiritual maturity comes with the promise of the agape love of the Father for those who agape love the Son. All references in the Scripture passage below refer to agape love:

The one who loves me will be loved by my Father, and I too will love them and show myself to him. If anyone loves me, he will obey my teaching. My Father will love him, and we will come to him and make our home with him. (John 14:21-24)

Agape love is not only our sanctification but our glorification. Without sanctification, we cannot be transformed, and without transformation, we cannot be glorified. Apostle Paul concluded:

The sufferings of this present time are not worth comparing with the glory that is going to be revealed in us. (Romans 8:18)

When Christ who is your life appears, then you also will appear with him in glory. (Colossians 3:4)

Beloved, we are God's children now, and what we will be has not yet appeared; but we know that when he appears we shall be like him, because we shall see him as he is. (1 John 3:2)

But our citizenship is in heaven, and from it we await a Savior, the Lord Jesus Christ, who will transform our lowly body to be like his glorious body. (Philippians 3:20–21)

Believers on this side of history, when the giving of the Holy Spirit had already happened, are without excuse. We, who have Jesus' words, the Holy Scripture, and the Holy Spirit, can understand and acquire this amazing agape love. How do we, then, measure our own growth in agape love?

Task: In light of the discussion on agape love, reread 1 Corinthians 13. This time, instead of reading the word "love," substitute it with "My agape love for Jesus." For example, "My agape love for Jesus never fails." Pay attention to the statements and consider how they might not fully represent your current agape love for Jesus, similar to the experience of the Apostle Peter in John 21:15-19. You might realize that, like Apostle Paul, your love for Jesus may be more at the "phileo" (brotherly) level. What will you do to change that? Share your thoughts.

_____

_____

_____

_____

_____

The references to agape love for Jesus that do not genuinely reflect an "agape" level of love for Him are the areas still under the control of the old, undead flesh. These must be renounced, brought to the cross, and crucified so that the new, Christ-like nature will be inscribed as your permanent, holy character.

Humanity was made in love. Humanity was made to love. It is a divinely imparted capacity that mirrors the love of the Creator. When not fulfilled, it leaves a gaping hole, a void in the soul; it sickens the human spirit. How are we to love then? Believers in Christ don't love as the world loves. Apostle Paul sets the standard in 1 Corinthians 13.

If I speak in the tongues of men or of angels, but do not have love, I am only a resounding gong or a clanging cymbal. If I have the gift of prophecy and can fathom all mysteries and all knowledge, and if I have a faith that can move mountains, but do not have love, I am nothing. If I give all I possess to the poor and surrender my body to the flames, but do not have love, I gain nothing. Love is patient, love is kind. It does not envy, it does not boast, it is not proud. It is not rude, it is not self-seeking, it is not easily angered, it keeps no record of wrongs. Love does not delight in evil but rejoices with the truth. It always protects, always trusts, always hopes, always perseveres. Love never fails. But where there are prophecies, they will cease; where there are tongues, they will be stilled; where there is knowledge, it will pass away. For we know in part and we prophesy in part, but when perfection comes, the imperfect disappears. When I was a child, I talked like a child, I thought like a child, I reasoned like a child.

When I became a man, I put the childish ways behind me. Now we see but a poor reflection as in a mirror; then we shall see face to face. Now I know in part; then I shall know fully, even as I am fully known. And now these three remain: faith, hope and love. But the greatest of these is love. (1 Corinthians 13)

Raham Agape Love—Sanctification

Salvation—Peace Like a River

Sanctification—Love Like a Spring of Living Water

Apostle Paul describes what divinely imparted agape love looks like (1 Corinthians 13). The finger of God inscribed on a tablet of stone the conditions for attaining this love—the Ten Commandments (Exodus 31:18). Jesus put the Law of God and the human capacity for agape love together, explaining that only through obedience to His commandments can we attain it. The entire Law of God is hinged on two commandments.

> 'Love the Lord your God with all your heart and with all your soul and with all your mind.' The second is like it: 'Love your neighbor as yourself.' All the Law and the Prophets hang on these two commandments. (Matthew 22:37-40)

God is love. God is agape (1 John 4:7-21). The Law of God breathes love. Meeting the righteous requirements of the Law of God comes with a reward—love, the agape kind. This reward is not the agape love with which God loves us. God's love is given, regardless of whether one is aware of it and accepts it. What is acquired through obedience to the Law of God is our capacity to love unconditionally, as God does. This way, we can love God back with the same measure He loves us. Because God is agape, we become agape also. This imparted agape love enables us to love our neighbor, even our enemy. This is the love Apostle Paul describes in 1 Corinthians 13. One cannot attain this kind of love apart from the Law of God. Apostle Paul pleads with the Ephesians,

> Be imitators of God, therefore, as dearly loved children and live a life of love [agape] just as Christ loved [agape] us and gave himself up for us as a fragrant offering and sacrifice to God. (Ephesians 5:1-2)

Question: As a believer, have I achieved the standards of agape love?

_____

_____

Many questions arise: Is it too high of a standard for the ordinary person to attain agape love? How do I meet the righteous requirements of the Law of God and attain this amazing agape love? The apostle who was the closest to Jesus, John, learned from Him the very truth of this divinely imparted agape love, so he passed it down to us:

Dear friends, let us love one another, for love comes from God. Everyone who loves has been **born** of God and **knows** God. Whoever does not love does not know God, because God is love. This is how God showed his love among us: He sent his one and only Son into the world that we might live through him. This is love: not that we loved God, but that he loved us and sent his Son as an atoning sacrifice for our sins.

Dear friends, since God so loved us, we also ought to love one another. No one has ever seen God; but if we love one another, God lives in us and his love is made complete in us.

We know that we live in him and he in us because he has given us his Spirit. And we have seen and testify that the Father has sent his Son to be the Savior of the world.

If anyone acknowledges that Jesus is the Son of God, God lives in him and he in God. And so we know and rely on the love God has for us.

God is love. Whoever lives in love lives in God, and God in him. In this way, love is made complete among us so that we will have confidence on the day of judgment because in this world we are like him. There is no fear in love. But perfect love drives out fear, because fear has to do with punishment. The one who fears is not made perfect in love.

We love because he first loved us. Whoever claims to love God yet hates a brother or sister is a liar. If one says, "I love God," yet hates his brother, he is a liar. For anyone who does not love their brother, whom he has seen, cannot love God, whom he has not seen. And he has given us this command: Whoever loves God must also love his brother.

(1 John 4:7-21, emphasis added)

In the above passage, Apostle John speaks specifically of agape love. He distinguishes between "being **born** of God and to **know** God." Everyone who wants to acquire this divine agape love must:

1) be **born** again— "born of God " and

2) **know** God personally, having a fellowship with Him—"to know God." The first condition refers to the salvation experience of a believer, and the second condition refers to sanctification that transforms the believer in the image of Christ. Jesus explained the **first** condition to a teacher of the Law, Nicodemus, twice,

> I tell you the truth, no one can see the kingdom of God unless he is born again. ... I tell you the truth, no one can enter the kingdom of God unless he is born of water and the Spirit. Flesh gives birth to flesh, but the Spirit gives birth to spirit. (John 3:3,5)

Jesus explained the **second** condition of sanctification to the woman at the well (John 4:5-30).

> Jesus answered her, "If you knew the gift of God and who it is that asks you for a drink, you would have asked him, and he would have given you living water." ... But whoever drinks of the water I give him shall never thirst. Indeed, the water I give

him will become in him a spring of water welling up to eternal life. (John 4:10,14)

The **first** teaching, to be born again, refers to one defined point in time when a person makes a decision to accept Jesus as God and Messiah and is saved. At that time, the Holy Spirit indwells the person.

The Spirit himself testifies with our spirit that we are God's children. (Romans 8:16)

The sign of the spiritual transaction of salvation is the **peace** of God, which surpasses all understanding (Philippians 4:7). This is the **peace like a river**, described by the Prophet Isaiah (Isaiah 48:18; 66:12-13). The **second** teaching, to know God, is a longer process through which the imparted power of the Holy Spirit enables the believers to shed off their old self with the old practices of the flesh and grow in the image of Christ (Galatians 5:24). This is the spring of living water Jesus and Prophet Jeremiah spoke about, referencing the state of **sanctification** (John 4:5-30; Jeremiah 2:13). **The hallmark of salvation is peace like a river; the hallmark of sanctification is the spring of living water**.

Because God lives in us, His agape love is made complete in us (1 John 4:12). Prophet Isaiah prophesied about this wonderful gift of God,

With joy, you will draw water from the wells of salvation. (Isaiah 12:3-5)

At the Festival of Tabernacles, Jesus stood at the temple courts, teaching about salvation and sanctification, and many believed in Him as the promised Messiah.

If anyone is thirsty, let him come to me and drink. Whoever believes in me, as the Scripture has said, streams of living water will flow from within him. (John 7:37,38)

The above texts describe the state of sanctification of a believer. The sign that this spiritual transaction has occurred is the impartation of God's divine agape love, which has now become an eminent part of a believer's character.

God is the well of salvation and the living water that sustains life into eternity with Him. **Peace is God's stamp of salvation. Raham or Agape love is God's stamp of sanctification.** Peace is granted upon salvation. Agape love is acquired with sanctification. Salvation positions us on the narrow road, but there is a critical qualifier that allows entry through the narrow gate into eternity with God (Matthew 7:13;14). On the narrow road, we must be transformed from glory to glory (2 Corinthians 3:18) into the image of Christ. Jesus called us to grow into the perfection of our Heavenly Father (Matthew 5:48). This is the process of sanctification. It is God's will that we should be sanctified (1 Thessalonians 4:3) and attain His agape love.

Apostle Paul narrates his own journey on the narrow road of sanctification. His ultimate victory of the Spirit over the flesh enabled him to describe the true nature of agape love.

I do not understand what I do. For what I want to do I do not do, but what I hate I do. And if I do what I do not want to do, I agree that the law is good. As it is, it is no longer I myself who do it, but it is sin living in me. I know that nothing good lives in me, that is, in my sinful nature. For I have the desire to do what is good, but I cannot carry it out.

For what I do is not the good I want to do; no, the evil I do not want to do—this I keep on doing. Now if I do what I do not want to do, it is no longer I who do it, but it is sin living in me that does it.

So I find this law at work: When I want to do good, evil is right there with me. For in my inner being I delight in God's law; but I see another law in the members of my body, waging war against the law of my mind and making me a prisoner of the law of sin at work within my members. What a wretched man I am! Who will rescue me from this body of death? Thanks be to God—through Jesus Christ our Lord!

So then, I myself in my mind am a slave to God's law, but in my sinful nature a slave to the law of sin. (Romans 7:15-20)

The only way to nullify the power of the "law of sin" is to condemn the sinful flesh to death on the cross. Apostle Paul triumphs in the victory over his old flesh, being crucified with Christ and yet much alive with Christ living in him (Galatians 2:20). Upon sanctification, we discard the old practices of the flesh, incompatible with the Kingdom of God, and clothe ourselves with His divine nature.

> Put off your old self, which is being corrupted by its deceitful
> desires; to be made new in the attitude of your minds, and to
> put on the new self, created to be like God in true
> righteousness and holiness. (Ephesians 4:22b-23)

Only by attaining Christ's new nature can one exhibit His divine agape love. Only then can one love God with the same love He loves us, and we can love our neighbor, even our enemy. When we reach this point of our journey, we have met the two requirements of the Law—to love God and to love the neighbor. This is the divine agape love made available to all who believe and sanctify themselves. Without the transformative presence of the Holy Spirit to cause us to agape love God and our neighbor, our natural love "is like a morning cloud, like the dew that goes early away" (Hosea 6:4).

The divinely imparted agape love contains phileo and eros. Eros, however, does not always contain agape or phileo. This is the watershed partition between love and casual, uncommitted sex: It is divinely to love with sexual passion with the full intent to procreate and, in return, create more agape love. It is humanly, though, to have sex just for the sole purpose of experiencing the divine gift of love. The first is the lifeline of a relationship divinely assigned to the office of marriage. The second is the dry line of a "liberated" relationship that starts and ends with pleasure—with no eternal benefits. The first brings the promised blessings (Deuteronomy 28); the second triggers the associated curses (Deuteronomy 29). This is the law of reaping and sowing in full display (Galatians 6:7-8).

Raham Agape Love and Trauma

The call for agape love might seem unattainable to believers who have experienced traumatic events such as abuse, violence, neglect, or betrayal. Yet, they are still expected to meet the two key commandments of God's Law: To love the Lord your God with all your heart, and with all your soul, and with all your mind, and to love your neighbor as yourself (Matthew 22:37,39).

First, we must validate the understanding that these individuals, having suffered the abuse, are in a much more difficult position when asked to love their neighbor, especially if the neighbor is the perpetrator causing the traumatic experience. And yet, the requirement of the Law of God to love the neighbor is not negated for the trauma victim. Despite the circumstances, God has not waived the righteous requirements of the Law. However, has not left the suffering believer to face their struggles alone; He provided help.

> The law was brought in so that the trespass might increase.
> But where sin increased, grace increased all the more.
> (Romans 5:20)

It is recognizably difficult, specifically for the victims of sexual abuse, to be tasked with displaying agape love toward the abuser. The severity of the trauma might have hindered the ability for an adequate response. When emotions are rampantly high, they tend to override reasoning, especially emotions connected with sexual violence. Overcoming this hindrance requires understanding how the act of sexual violence and the consequential trauma trigger the Law of God, turning the victim into a lawbreaker. The victims are innocent, involuntary participants in the violent act against God's Law. Their involvement doesn't trigger the curses associated with the act of sexual violence, but their response toward the perpetrator does. The enemy uses the natural response of hatred, animosity, rage, anger, bitterness, and ultimately unforgiveness against the victims, putting them in a position of lawbreakers. The Scripture tells us that,

> Anyone who hates his brother is a murderer, and you know
> that no murderer has eternal life residing in him. (1 John 3:15)

The enemy has used the situation to place the victim from a spiritual state of innocence to a state of guilt, from life to death, because,

> Whoever hates his brother is in the darkness and walks
> around in the darkness; he does not know where he is going
> because the darkness has blinded him. (1 John 2:11)

The Scripture also calls the victim to forgive the perpetrator. To forgive the offender is a part of the Lord's prayer.

> And forgive us our debts, as we also have forgiven our debtors.
> … But if you do not forgive men their sins, your Father will
> not forgive your sins. (Matthew 6:12,15)

The victims are held to an even higher standard, making the task desperately unachievable: Not only to forgive but also to love the offender with agape love.

> You have heard that it was said, 'Love your neighbor and hate
> your enemy.' But I tell you: Love your enemies and pray for
> those who persecute you, that you may be sons of your Father
> in heaven. (Matthew 5:43)

Yes, the victim is placed in the impossible position to love the violent offender with no other love but agape love. Holding to anger and hatred gives the victim some sense of control over the perpetrator. Holding to anger and hatred, however, is like venom spat towards the offender but swallowed by the victim. The victim's turmoil doesn't affect the perpetrator but consumes the victim, affecting their physical, emotional, mental, and spiritual well-being.

Yes, "the enemy has done this," Jesus said, referring to the evil in this world. (Matthew 13:28). Indeed, the enemy has deceived us once again, ensuring the destruction of both the perpetrator and the victim. The enemy succeeds if it convinces the victim that holding onto hatred and anger is justified to seek retribution for the offender and justice for the victim.

God has defeated the enemy and his schemes. He redeemed us from the curse of the Law. He provided a path of purification and righteousness for the victim. It is the narrow road that only a few will find (Matthew 7:13-14). The journey on the narrow road, as discussed earlier in session six, requires completing these basic biblical steps: 1) renounce the practices of old flesh, such as unforgiveness, anger, and hatred; 2) nail these on the cross; 3) wash in His blood; 4) be filled with the Spirit of the living God. Throughout this process, continually praise God for the provision He has planned since the beginning of time (1 Peter 1:20) to rescue you from the curse of the Law and the enemy of our soul.

Applying this approach for spiritual restoration is an act of faith: The old has gone, the new has come (2 Corinthians 5:17). The new self is being clothed with the new divine nature of our Savior, Christ Jesus. This is the process of sanctification and transformation in the image of Christ, through which the victim attains God's agape love.

Only through the cross can the victim experience renewed joy in giving and receiving agape love. Only through the cross does the impossible task of agape love the perpetrator become possible. We don't have the capacity to love our neighbor as ourselves (Mark 12:31). We don't have the capacity to love the perpetrator. We have a great capacity to hate the perpetrator. Christ's indwelling in us, however, changes this dynamic. Because He lives in me, it is not my agape love but His agape love that lives in me, making me capable of agape love, even the perpetrator. What was impossible in the old flesh is now a reality through the indwelling of the Holy Spirit. The agape love toward the perpetrator **manifests as empathy** for the lost soul, steeped in sin. If you have empathy toward your perpetrator, you have attained agape love.

Glorification—Final Consummation of EHAD

In the garden of Gethsemane, Jesus prayed for Himself, His disciples, and all who would come after them (John 17). His final prayer includes two key themes related to glorification:

1) The unity of the disciples: Jesus desires that His disciples be ONE/EHAD just as He and the Father are ONE/EHAD (John 17:11, 21-23, 26).

2) Glorification as a final consummation of becoming ONE/EHAD with God (John 17:5,17-19; 22-24).

Upon His ascension, Jesus is glorified in God's presence with the glory He had before the world began (John 17:5). Jesus has given us the same glory that the Father gave Him, that we may be EHAD, just as Jesus and the Father are EHAD (John 17:22). One day, we will see Jesus in His glory. This same glory will transform us into His likeness of divine righteousness and will be our glory because Jesus bestowed it upon us (John 17:22).

The final chapter of our redemption is glorification. It is the culmination and the finalization of our sanctification. From the moment of salvation, the indwelling of the Holy Spirit begins the transformation into the image of Christ. The work is not finished until we enter eternity with God, where our sanctification is perfected.

There is a chasm between the righteousness of Christ on one side and the righteousness of a most righteous person, like the Apostle Paul, on the other side. There is still an existing abyss between the sinless Jesus and the most righteous, unglorified person, like the Apostle Paul. Upon justification, we are saved, and through the work of the Holy Spirit, we are sanctified. However, it is only when we enter eternity in the presence of Jesus that we will fully conform to His sinless nature, free from sin. This is the consummation of our sanctification. It starts on earth, but it is perfected in heaven. This is our glorification. It is a journey from the Great Commission (Matthew 28:16–20) to joining the great multitude in heaven that no one could count, from every nation, tribe, people, and language, standing before the throne and before the

Lamb (Revelation 7:9). Until then, we must fight the good fight, finish the race, and keep the faith. In store for us is the crown of righteousness, which the Lord, the righteous Judge, will award to us on that day (2 Timothy 4:7-8).

EHAD with GOD

REFLECTION—Week Nine

Reflection 1: Give Him 5—practicing God's presence (see description on pages 41 and 63 under "Deep calls to deep" section)

Reflection 2: Daily confession and repentance in prayer to Christ—our high priest; crucify the flesh, wash with the blood, fill with the Holy Spirit (page 13)

Reflection 3: The Story of Alma Bella—Compassion and Empathy

The Story of Alma Bella[17]

The Surgery, Year 2004, Los Angeles, California

"I don't want anybody to hold me. Not even you, Victoria. I don't want to see anybody. I don't need anybody now. Why is everybody circling around? Why the hassle? I'm fine. Can you just leave me alone? Get away from me, you all! Leave me alone, alone, alone...." My mind was screaming at the many doctors and nurses hovering over my hospital bed, but all they could see was my "crying." Don't they know that I can't cry? Don't they see that I have no tears?

The lights were painfully bright, streaming in a cold-white flow from above, exposing me to all those strangers. They shuttled between the armada of medical equipment, and it made me sick. My eyes hurt, but I was afraid to close them. I was scared I would faint again. The surgery was over. I knew I was in the intensive care unit.

---

[17] Excerpt from Shaynah Neshama, *All Shall Be Well*, Tree of Life Publishing House, 2006.

It was over! Why was I so scared? No, I was terrified. I dreaded losing my life. I was horrified that I might die. I didn't care about my life, but not at that moment, not when my Mama was on her way to see me, probably very close to the hospital. My aunt said that she had told her about my surgery. My aunt said that she would come with my Mama to be with me at the hospital. I did not see my aunt when they took me in. Neither did I see my Mama. My Mama was not there when I woke up in intensive care. My aunt said she would come. Oh, Mama...you didn't come to be with me.

"I don't care about all of you here. I don't want doctors. I don't want nurses. I don't want social workers! Even you, Victoria, I don't want you now. All of you, just leave me..." With all the strength of my mind, I shouted in despair, "I don't care if I die now. My Mama is what I want...I want my Mama...but she is gone. Where are you, Mama? I hurt so badly, Mama. It hurts, Mama,...It hurts.... Where are you to hold me now? Mama, hold me, Mama.... Tell me that you will never leave me again.... Come back, Mama... I'll be a good girl, Mama....Oh, Mama...Mama...Mama. Where are you, Mama? Oh, Mama... Mama...Mama..., come back...!"

The one I wanted most at that moment had vanished from my life long ago. How much I missed her presence around that hospital bed! I wanted everybody to leave and my Mama to come, sit next to me, hold me, and rock me in her arms, close to her heart. If she could just have come and held me, I would have been okay. But my Mama did not come. She did not hold me. She did not rock me. She, indeed, had vanished.

I was alone! A lonely leaf that had been taken by a sudden surge of wind and brought to an icy cold place. Like that leaf that had no chance of seeing the spring come, so was I with no chance to see a motherly love in my life. On that hospital bed, while a powerful fluorescent light glared at me, my heart entered a long, pitch-dark night; while a multitude of people swirled around me, I felt painfully alone. Alone! I was alone! Alone in the cold, alone in the dark, without my Mama.... Abandoned!

All these long years, I had thought my Mama somehow would come back and take us all home. For a long time, I had clung to the hope that she would finally relent and return after being away for so many years. There was no hope anymore. At that moment, then and there, the cold fact that my Mama had abandoned me hit me with tremendous power. My heart sank inside my chest so deeply I was sure if the nurse had looked at me at that moment, she would have seen the ugly hole that formed under my thin hospital gown. Rising from that internal hole was a gigantic wave of pain. Deep roaring, "Alone! Alone! Alone!" set waves of uncontrollable trembling through my body. Cruel mocking, "Abandoned! Abandoned! Abandoned!" began to gnaw away at what was left of my battered world of sorrow.

"Mama...Mama...Mama...." I fought back the ugly tentacles of pain that suffocated me, but my attempt was like the effort of a single drop against a giant wave that ultimately absorbed it. My body was failing me; I could not move. My mouth was failing me; I could not shout. I willed my mind to scream, and I heard the scream of my heart instead. A wild howl jabbed at my sides, my body cramping in two. Like a sleeping beast that had been hibernating for a long time, the pain in my heart awoke with the realization that I had been completely abandoned. So was the howling of my heart. I was sure the attending nurses heard it because they all began panicking around me. More needles, more injections, more tubes, and the awful smell of antiseptic until all began to fade. The nurses floated away, the noises grew distant, and the lights above dimmed. I fell into that blur of images, and light and weightlessly floated away along with everything around me.

The pain had been my companion since my birth. With my first cry, along with air, my lungs must have filled with the contempt my mother had when she first looked at me. On the first day of my life, my mother's first touch was stamped with disdain, not love. I was her firstborn child, but instead of joy, my aunt said, I had brought her only problems. My mother was sixteen then, and I had no legitimate father.

The bitterness that poisoned my mother's life had also poisoned my life right from the beginning. Hatred consumed my mother and reduced her to a mere day-to-day "moving along" existence. I remember the long hours watching her prostrate on the bare floor, crying louder and louder. I would become so scared that I'd try to climb on or sit next to her, but she would angrily toss me away.

In time, I learned that cuddling up in the darkness in the furthest corner was the right thing to do. So, I tried to be invisible. From the dark, I watched how those scary needles pierced my mom's arm and then rolled onto the floor with a metallic clatter.

When her body had fallen in a heap, an amorphous mass in the middle of the room, then I knew it was safe for me to come out and be with my Mama. It was dark and frighteningly silent, but I loved those moments when I could lie beside my Mama. I could touch her beautiful face and play with her soft hair. I would take her arm, put it around my shoulders, and kiss each of her slender, pale fingers one by one. When it was cold, I dragged out a heavy blanket and tucked both of us beneath its rough cover. I treasured those quiet moments with my Mama, and I would not give them up for anything, not even for a big, out-of-the-oven, hot slice of pizza that would have quieted the spasms of hunger rumbling in my empty stomach.

Coming the second time out of anesthesia was no better than the first. The grief that had exacerbated my post-surgical condition earlier threatened to overrun my fragile state of heart again. A familiar voice encouraged me to try harder to wake up, but that voice had less control over me than the pain welling up inside. The brightness of the lights still stung my eyes, but at least the hassled nurses were gone, and the annoying beeping of the many machines around my bed had subsided. A lonely silhouette leaned over me as I tried to adjust my eyes to the blinding light. Victoria stood beside my bed, saying something I could not hear, but I could feel her fingers lightly stroking my hand.

"Bella, Bella," she exclaimed when she saw me coming out from the sedative influence of the drugs, "it is all over, Bella. The doctor said it all went well. My brave Bella! The doctor said that now we can go home."

"Home? I have no home, Victoria. You know. I don't want to go back to that foster home. Can't you take me with you to your home? Can you? Please, Victoria, say that you can take me with you." Victoria has always been nice to me, doing many things a mother would do. She was so beautiful, and everybody liked her. If I could choose where I wanted to go, without hesitation, I would prefer to go with Victoria.

"My dear Bella, I wish I could take you home, but you know how many rules are in the system? I don't want to break them, Bella, and you don't want me to either. What I can do is promise you to take you out this weekend. What do you say? Where would you wanna go?"

"With you, to your home," I said dryly, cooled off by the fast calculations happening in my head. "It's only Thursday night now, Victoria, and you wouldn't come until Saturday, yeah?"

"That means only one day, Bella, just one day."

She unsuccessfully tried to provoke a positive emotion in me.

"One day and two nights, Victoria, is long, very long...." I was powerless and like a canary bound by a cage, so was I bound to lose her. I knew that very soon, she would take me to the foster home, and then she would be gone.

"Nights we sleep, Bella, and they go fast," she tried to reason, but her arguments did not cheer me up.

"You sleep, Victoria. I don't. Nightmares haunt me, you know. They seem to leave me alone only when you're around. Could you take me with you, Victoria? Be my Mama."

Tears ran down Victoria's beautiful face. She did not try to hide them. She never did. When she first came to visit me at the foster home, she could not stop crying. Her tears flowed and flowed while I told her what had happened to me. She had said that from that moment on, she would cry with me when I was sad and laugh with me when I would be happy. And she did. There had been many times when we laughed together, but there had been more times when she cried alone. I couldn't cry. I felt the pain squeezing me to death, but tears would not come out of my eyes.

"You need to rest, Bella. We will have time to talk about these things another time. You had a hard day today, but it's all over now. I have a surprise for you, Bella. It is a little thing, but perfect for a brave girl like you."

Victoria always found ways to route our conversations differently. But this time, I did not want to let her go. I had become very crafty in finding ways to make her stay longer at the foster home. No matter how hard I worked to keep her with me, the time always came when she had to leave. Something very bright always left with her. Right then, I did not want to lose her bright presence, not after that treacherous day of my surgery.

"Victoria, did I cry during the surgery or after that?" I asked Victoria as the nurses pulled the long curtains at both sides of my bed, scarcely giving us privacy from the other two patients in the room. I wanted to know if I had cried while under anesthesia.

"No, Bella, you did not cry. I saw no tears on your face, but I saw something much more painful." Hesitance clouded Victoria's face. She realized that she had said more than she had intended.

"What is it, Victoria? You know I can take it. What is it you saw?" I pulled her by the arm, making her sit next to me.

"I saw your soul crying," she said, almost whispering, slowly accenting each word.

"My soul?" I was puzzled by Victoria's words. As with showing her tears, Victoria was not ashamed about her faith either. God, she had said, loved her, and that same God also loved me. I couldn't understand how someone like God could love me, and I didn't feel it. When Victoria said she loved me, I knew it was true because I felt it; she made me feel it. At that time, though, I knew nothing about the "soul" business. Simple logic kept my interest. If such a good person like Victoria was so keen on spiritual matters, I thought it worth finding out why.

"My dear Bella, your soul was crying. I saw all the sorrow and pain locked inside your heart and soul. Your Mama and Franky are gone, but the pain they caused is not gone." When Victoria saw that I remained puzzled at her words, she continued, "You see, Bella, the tears are like channels through which the poisonous substance of pain is released. When we cry, the poison leaves our hearts. We cry, and the pain lessens. When we don't cry, the pain remains locked inside, piling up like a huge mountain, and the bigger it gets, the more poisonous it becomes." After a moment of hesitation, Victoria looked at me with deep concern in her eyes and said, "When you came out of the surgery, I saw your mountain of pain. Bella, I saw your soul crying."

I still couldn't understand what Victoria was telling me. Many times during our therapy sessions, Victoria kept encouraging me that crying was okay and that I shouldn't feel embarrassed, but I told her that I couldn't cry. I had my own explanation for my inability to produce tears.

"I guess a certain amount of tears is ascribed to each individual to use throughout their lifetime, and when all the tears have been released, the eyes just dry out."

"And when do you suppose you have reached your lifetime tears limit?" Victoria had asked.

"When my Mama left us with Franky. The belt in his hand felt much heavier on my back. Tears made him mad, so I learned to hold them back." I explained, but I wondered if Victoria could ever understand what life with Franky had been like.

"Did Junior and Alicia learn that also?" Victoria asked about my half-brother and half-sister. She was sincere in her efforts to make sense of the severe abuse we had suffered, but I doubted if it would ever be possible for her, or anyone else, to comprehend it.

"No, they were too little. Sometimes, they cried so much and wanted our Mama. But that made Franky so mad that he had his belt burning on my back over and over again." I paused momentarily and added, "You know that Alicia and Junior are his children ... but Franky is not my father."

"His anger was more often directed at you than to them, yes?"

"Yes, but he turned on them, too." I couldn't stand watching Franky hurting Junior and Alicia. They were so tiny and so helpless. It was after one of those beatings that a teacher noticed Junior's bruises and called me to the principal's office, as well.

The nurse in charge poked her head through the folds of the heavy curtain. "It is time for you, Mama, to take Bella home." She waved the discharge papers clutched in her hand, saying, "I need to give you some instructions, and I need some signatures, and you are ready to go." The nurse took Victoria aside behind the curtain. From my bed, I could hear the thorough instructions given to Victoria about my post-surgical care.

"I didn't know you were a social worker," the nurse said after seeing Victoria's signature on the papers. "We all thought that you were the mother," the nurse's apologetic voice muffled by the steady clamor in the room.

"I am still family," I heard Victoria say, and hope swelled up in my heart.

It was dark when they rolled me out in the wheelchair and helped me get in Victoria's car—twelve long hours had passed since I had entered the hospital for outpatient surgery that morning. A wide bandage was tightly secured on my head.

"How will I go to school like this, Victoria?" I complained, pointing to the bandage and looking in the car mirror, hoping to find a solution.

"You are not going to school until Tuesday, Bella. The doctor wants to change the dressing on Monday, and he said that they would remove that big one and leave you with a tiny bandage. It will be under your long hair, unseen."

Having even a small part of my beautiful hair shaved was not comforting. I flaunted my hair before my friends in school. Since my detention in foster care, I had let it grow and worn it loose. It had been a good cover for the ugly bump steadily growing on the back of my head.

I had little concern for it, but it worried Victoria when I mentioned it. She said that it was probably connected to my fainting episodes. I had grown up with those episodes that could happen any time, day or night. Junior and Alicia were so accustomed to seeing me passing out and coming back into consciousness twenty minutes later that they had learned to wait patiently for me when that would happen.

Victoria, though, appeared very concerned and kept asking me if I remembered ever hitting my head in the past. I couldn't make any connection between an old head injury and my episodes of fainting, but by Victoria's reaction, I understood it was very important for her to know. At first, I couldn't remember hitting myself, but later, I told her what had happened once when I was very little. It was one of the stories Victoria had not heard yet.

I hated all those big men who kept coming to our apartment. Their shouts and loud laughter frightened me. I hid in the dark closet, and from there, my fear would grow into a nightmare because of all the scary things those men did to my Mama. At first, I thought she was hurt, but that was the only time I saw my Mama happy and laughing. The more she laughed, the more I cried.

Once, she dragged me out of the closet, very upset at me. With fists and curses, she threw herself furiously at me. Angrily, she stuck a threatening finger in my face and said that if I didn't stop crying, she would tell the men to do the same things to me. I was terrified. I wanted to stop crying, but my Mama kept pulling my hair and pounding her fists. I hurt so much that I not only continued crying but I began screaming. The high pitch of my loud protest infuriated my mother further. She threw me against the wall and began banging my head against it.

I don't know what hurt more—the blows on my head or the words she shouted at me. She said that I was her burden, and that she hated me, and that she should have killed me when I was still in her tummy. I didn't want to hear all that, but I couldn't run from my Mama. Then, all at once, everything went quiet in my head. My eyes dimmed, and my ears grew dull to her words. I didn't know what had happened, but when I could see again, I was in my mother's arms. She was rocking me, squeezing me tightly, and crying loudly, "My baby, wake up, baby, wake up. I am sorry, mijita[18], I am sorry, mi niñita[19], come back. I promise I will not do this again. I will be a good mamá. I am sorry, baby. Come back, mi bella[20], mi alma bella[21]...mi bellisima[22]...."

She continued sobbing for a long time, even when I regained consciousness. "What did I do to my baby? How could I do this to my child? Oh, damn me...I could have killed her.... Oh, no...I am an animal. No, even the animals don't kill their babies. What am I? Sweetie, forgive Mama, say that you forgive Mama. I will try to be a better mama to you. Forgive my hands for bruising your little body. Forgive my mouth for saying awful things. Can you forgive Mama, baby?"

I was crying then, but not because my head was pounding with pain. I knew my Mama loved me. I wanted my Mama to love me. She hadn't wanted to do all this to me. It was all my fault; I should have kept quiet. I should have been stronger and not cried.

"Oh, Mama...I am going to be a good girl," I said, but my voice was too weak to be heard over her loud monologue. "I love you, mama; I am not going to cry again, I promise." I was unsure that my Mama had heard me, so I repeated it, louder and again, until her eyes finally fixed on me.

"Mi niñita, mi Alma Bella...I love you, I love you, I love you...." My Mama kissed me all over, her hands probing up and down my body. With feverish

---

[18] Spanish for my little daughter

[19] Spanish for my little girl

[20] Spanish for beautiful

[21] Spanish for beautiful soul

[22] Spanish for my beautiful little girl

eyes, she examined me for signs of visible damage. "You are okay, mi hija[23], yes? You look okay. Does something hurt you? Can you stretch your arms? Good...." She exhaled loudly in relief when she saw that nothing was broken. "Good...very good," she laughed nervously. Then, with brisk strokes, she moved up my body to examine my head.

"Oh..." I cried, but my cry did not relieve the pain she touched caused. Then, I saw her dark brows closing together high on her forehead. I regretted being such a crybaby. I knew she was not happy. I did not want to disappoint my Mama, not then and there, not when she had just told me that she loved me and that she would not hit me anymore. "No, Mama, just a little," I lied. "It hurts but only a little, Mama, but I am a big girl now, and I will not pay attention, and it will go away. It will not hurt me anymore, Mama."

My mother was not listening to me anymore. Her attention was entirely fixed on her outstretched hand, opened wide in front of her—covered with blood, my blood, smeared between her fingers. I was so scared when I saw the sudden disgust on my mother's face. I was not sure what evoked it, the sight of my blood or the repulsion she felt for me at that moment. In either case, I was bound to lose my Mama again.

"I know that you are a big girl, Bella. It is only a little scratch, a very small thing. Nothing is broken, Bella. We don't need a doctor here. Mama will take care of everything, mijita." My Mama kept talking sweetly while she cleaned the blood that had begun to dry, plastered on my hair.

Later, she went to McDonalds and got me a Happy Meal with a small toy inside. If a broken skull could secure me another hour sitting on my mother's lap and eating a McDonald Happy Meal, I would readily have chosen the same fate anytime again. I was thankful in my heart for that little incident because it diverted my mother's attention solely to me for the rest of the day.

---

[23] Spanish for my daughter

"We don't have to tell others about our little incident today, Bella." my mother whispered in my ear, indicating great importance. And all the matters of that day became a secret to which we silently agreed.

My mamma did not take me to the hospital, then. She was already gone when the episodes of fainting began. Franky did not think I needed medical attention, either. Victoria and the doctor, however, were so alarmed by the bump on my head that I was immediately scheduled for surgery. The doctor said that scar tissue had grown at the place of my injury and had to be removed. I still couldn't understand how that could be related to my fainting episodes, but I trusted Victoria and the doctor when they said it did.

The Interview

"What is your name, sweetheart?" asked the young woman with the long red-painted nails who had been diligently writing my information on a large sheet of paper. Her scratchy voice grated on me like her fingernails on that parched paper.

"Bella. My name is Alma Bella, ma'am," I answered, as my agitation grew with each question she asked.

"What a beautiful name!" she exclaimed with the trained intonation of a person who had dealt with children a lot, but her eyes remained on the papers.

"That's what it means. 'Bella' means 'beautiful,' " I said, "and 'Alma' means 'soul.' A Beautiful Soul," I added.

My simple explanation always seemed to stir people's interest, as it did with this woman.

"Beautiful Soul!" she exclaimed again, but this time, she looked at me from under the thin-framed glasses that had fallen low on her nose. She studied me, repeating my name as if trying to see if its sound and meaning befitted the appearance of the small, frightened child curled up on the chair in front of her.

"I can't see your soul, but I see that you are beautiful. Everybody can see that," she said, apparently satisfied with the results of her observations. "Well,

Alma Bella, I think we have covered everything necessary. Mr. Walton and Ms. Gomez will be with you shortly."

At the recognition of Mr. Walton's name, my heart began racing. Victoria had told me that he was the dependency investigator assigned to my case and would ask me questions about Franky.

"It won't be any different from the time you first reported it to the school and the police, Bella," Victoria had explained to me when I asked why I had to tell that man about Franky also. "He is not a policeman or counselor; he works with the court. The judge has sent him to find out what had happened to you, Junior, and Alicia. Are you afraid?" she asked.

"No," I answered, but I lied. Deep inside, I was torn between telling the truth, as Victoria always urged me to do, and my promise to Junior and Alicia.

Suddenly, I did not want to be there. I did not want to face another man again and tell him about Franky. I didn't want to tell anybody anymore what he did to me. How could anyone ever understand? And what good would that do me when Alicia and Junior were unhappy? Maybe they were right! Perhaps putting up with Franky was better than being in a foster home. It would probably not be that long before they treat us just like Franky did.

"Hello, Alma Bella!" A bearded middle-aged man interrupted my thoughts as he greeted me from the door, left half-open by the woman with the red-painted nails. "Alma Bella, yes? How do you like to be called, child?" he asked.

I shrugged my shoulders. I did not care what he called me. I did not want him to call me anything, anyway. I didn't want to be there. I did not want to talk to him. Why didn't Victoria come with me? I sighed.

"Hello! I am Ms. Gomez." A short woman wearing high heels and a tight, flowery dress followed the bearded man through the door and closed it behind her. "Bella," she said, "I thought you might be uncomfortable with some of the questions Mr. Walton would be asking. So, I came along with him to help you. I am with you now, not as a social worker, but more like girl-to-girl support. Do you understand?" She had come closer to me, pulled down one of the chairs stacked up in the back of the room, and sat across from me. When I remained silent, she added in Spanish, "If you are more comfortable talking in Spanish, mija, that would be just fine."

I did not want to talk! Not in English! Not in Spanish! Don't they get it? I did not want to talk, and I was not going to talk! The woman kept coming closer to me, lowering herself to look at me at my eye level. I felt as if I were being pushed back against a wall. I panicked. What did they all want from me? Why don't they go and ask Franky? For sure, he would not tell them anything. He said he would kill me if I did. I am dead-dead anyway!

"Do you remember, Bella, when your mom left Junior, Alicia, and you with Franky?" the bearded man asked when I remained silent. "What was life like for a young girl like you? You must have been like a mother to Alicia and Junior, yes?"

A mother for Alicia and Junior and a wife for Franky, I thought in my heart, but I said nothing. What did they know about a little girl forced to do all the laundry by hand instead of going out to play? I had to climb on a chair to reach the sink because the faucet was too high. What did they know about making a dinner for two toddlers from a "Cup of Noodles," two potatoes, and a carrot? What did they know about carrying baby Alicia, burning with a high fever, all the way to Tia Maria to get help? Franky was either gone or dead, drunk asleep. What did they know when, in his good moods, Franky would not beat me but pull me down alongside him on the bed and tell me that it was time to love each other as a good family does? How can they tell me they knew? Do they know that Franky's love hurt more than his other punishments? For Franky, it was a reward. Do they think of this as a reward also? Does this bearded man reward his children this way? How can he understand their pain, then?

"I understand your intimidation, Bella. I understand your pain. You have the right to be angry and refuse to talk." The woman in the flowery dress stroked my hand, but that did not open my mouth.

Does she really know my pain? Does she really know what pain is? I was boiling inside, but my emotional valve was tightly closed, refusing to let the steam of my pain, shame, and anger escape. Could she ever imagine what it was like for me, just a little girl, to be awakened during the night with yells and kicks, thrown in the bathtub, and ordered to stay there, my body submerged in cold water, until Franky's fury subsided? It was freezing cold. At times, I was losing it. My tears seemed to turn into icicles and crystallized on my bloodless cheeks. Everything inside turned dead cold. I felt like screaming my pain out, but Franky would have killed me before the neighbors heard my cry. I begged Franky. I begged him harder and harder, but that was my punishment, he said, for wetting my bed and wetting him while sleeping next to him. There were nights I was afraid to go to sleep because of those accidents that had begun to happen more often, not only at night but during the daytime, too. Does this woman really understand my pain? Does she really understand what the pain was?

The man and the woman kept talking, but I was far away, in a place where the painful memories turned into haunting shadows. I felt as if my entire body was shutting down. My mouth was not responsive. Neither were my eyes nor my ears. I could not hear what the bearded man and the woman in the flowery dress were saying to me. Their voices and figures seemed to fade away like the images of some distant characters in a slow-motion movie. My head was spinning. I wanted to run away from them. I wanted to hide, but there was nowhere to go. Their questions hammered away at the strength of my will to resist the painful memories of Franky. Even the wall I had first backed up against began crumbling behind me, leaving me with nothing to hold on to. I held on to that crumbling wall with the last traces of my strength, hoping that rescue would arrive. When the door opened, not rescue but the woman with the red-painted nails came in. She left a tray on the table and handed me a glass of water, saying something to me. Her mouth, colored with the same red she had on her nails, opened in what seemed a distorted smile. Terrified, I realized that my inner world of perceptions was painfully distorting images and sounds, causing everything my eyes fell on or my ears heard to appear ugly and distorted.

I heard the bearded man say, "When was the first time Franky touched you inappropriately, Bella?" A sudden distortion of his voice loomed at me with frightening dimensions. His face swelled, threatening to fill the entire room with its massive size and volume.

First time? Was there ever a first time? Was there ever a life without Franky? My memories were filled with him, my body scarred by him. Couldn't they see it? My soul was splintered with fear of him. Couldn't they feel it? Suddenly, the face of the bearded man took the shape of Franky's face; his voice began to sound like Franky's voice.

Franky's image came out fully alive from the dark closets of my mind, where I had been trying to keep him locked since our detention. He was coming at me, his eyes cracked open, looking intensely at me. He gathered my hair in his hand and pulled my head backward. I froze in anticipation of another of his punishments for something I did or should have done. He lowered his face to me, puckered his lips, and then backed up, laughing loudly. Toxic fumes of liquor and nicotine blasted from his mouth, making me hold my breath instinctively. I dared not show discontent. I just wondered why he had returned so early from work that day. Alicia and Junior were still with Tia Maria.

Franky, still laughing, took me in his arms and said he would show me how much he loved me. Franky had never before held me that way. His rough, stained-with-machine-oil hands that had pummeled me that same morning were now exploring my body with unknown excitement.

"I will teach you, mija, something only for big girls. It is time for Franky to teach you something good. It is time that Franky shows you the sweet part of life. Now relax, and you will see how you like what I will show you today."

Franky put me on his lap and feverishly moved his hands up and down my body. His touch was different from anything I had ever experienced before.

Nobody, not even my Mama, had ever shown me such affection as Franky did then. I stiffened in his arms, not knowing how to respond to his new "love."

"Relax, mija, just relax. Relax, mi linda[24]," Franky whispered huskily in my ear. "Kiss Franky, mija; show that you love me. I will show you how much I love you."

"Like you loved Mama?" I asked.

"Yes, mija, like Mama. But Mama is not here now, but you are. I show my love to you...."

I had watched silently in the dark many times when Mama and Franky loved each other this way. I was happy because they were happy and, for some time after that, they seemed to quarrel no more. Franky was giving that love to me now. At that moment, I wanted Franky to love me. He was my family. My Mama had left and had never come back. Probably, I thought, Franky was lonely too, and I wanted to give him my love.

I let Franky slip off my dress and panties...and then...it seemed that Franky lost his patience with me. His voice sounded muffled as if I was hearing it through the roaring of raging water, unclear and frightening. His breath quickened, and his eyes closed. He was not laughing anymore. His hands were not gentle on my body anymore. I heard my chest cracking under the pressure of his heavy body. A sharp pain ripped me from inside. There was no sound in the scream I cried out. There was no breath left in me to form that scream. An unknown pain entered my body; that enormous pain jolted my body, that cruel pain crippled my body, and that pain finally paralyzed my body. Franky was coming at me with full force with an ever-unceasing starvation; he threw himself at me violently.

"Mama...Mama...," I cried out, but my Mama was not there to take me away from Franky's hands. She was not there to protect me. I couldn't push Franky away from me. His face came at me, ugly and distorted, and took the shape of the bearded man.

---

[24] Spanish for my pretty girl

275

"Bella..., Bella...," the distorted image that resembled partly Franky and partly that bearded man was coming at me, calling my name; a monstrous creature from the order of gargoyles was stretching its hands towards me. The images and the sounds became so convoluted that my mind set my body for an immediate survival response.

"Don't touch me!" I screamed, fighting the images. "No, Franky! No!" My mind drifted between the reality of the office and the dark times and places I had suffered not long ago. The red-painted nails of the woman flashed before my eyes as she waved her arms to get my attention. Their color triggered memories of another red, the red of my blood trickling down from within me to the floor. I saw again those streams of blood that crawled down the drain and stained the bathtub with their bright red color, the same color as those red-painted nails.

"I am dying, Mama, I am dying, Mama...come, Mama...I don't want to die, Mama...," I cried, but Franky said Mama would not hear me. Nobody heard me. Nobody saw the rivers of blood, of my blood. Franky, like my Mama, said we did not need a doctor. Like my Mama, he said it would heal like a scratch on a puppy.

"Mama, oh, Mama...I hurt so much...why did you leave me? Mama... oh, Mama...come back...." I wanted my Mama, nothing else but my Mama. That day, the last brink of hope of having my Mama collapsed. I was just a little girl, only six years old, all alone against Franky and his horrifying punishments! I could not understand. How did the adults ever think of such cruel punishments for little kids and still call it love?

"It is okay, Bella," I heard the woman in the flowery dress say. "We don't have to talk today. It all seems very painful for you. You need to rest now. We can talk another time when you feel much stronger, okay?" Her words suddenly catapulted me away from the damaging memories of Franky.

"I lied," I said while the woman was still talking. "I lied," I repeated with a much stronger voice. They wanted me dismissed, and I could not let that happen. What was I going to tell Alicia and Junior? I feared that I had failed them. I could not stand their resentment anymore. Since I had told the school authorities about Franky, they had blamed me for our displacement. I could not understand why they would want to go back with Franky. After all the beatings they suffered? "I love him," Junior had said. "I love him, too," Alicia had said also. I guessed Franky was our only family, good or bad, but family.

Life with the Gonzalezes was quiet and clean. We had our own rooms and beds. With Franky, there was only one bunk bed. Junior and Alicia slept on the top, and Franky and I were on the bottom. With the Gonzalezes, we had clothes, shoes, and food—things we had never had with Franky. The Gonzalezes did not beat us, but they did not hug us either. At least on his good days, Franky had shown us some affection. Junior and Alicia missed those moments; I did not feel deprived of them at all. They believed that if I told the investigator I had lied about Franky, they would be allowed to return with him. I did not want to go back. I hoped that Victoria would somehow keep me with her.

"I lied," I said a third time, boldly looking into the eyes of the bearded man, the investigator. I became aware of other people who had filled the small office and had formed a tight circle around me. Their faces looked concerned, and their voices sounded troubled.

"Are you saying everything you ever said about Franky was not true? Is that correct, Bella?" the bearded man asked.

"I made it up," I said, barely holding myself together under the man's searching eyes.

Franky said I was good at lying and had learned it from him. He lied to the school many times about the reasons I would not show up for class or how I got my bruises. For that whole week, when the blood would not stop gushing out of me, Franky ordered me not to go to school. He told my teacher that I was sick with the flu. I also lied to my teacher when she asked me if I had improved. The bleeding never completely stopped because Franky never stopped. With time, the sight of my blood became a side effect of his "love," and nobody paid attention to it anymore. I learned to live with the pain and the sight of blood.

"So, it turns out that Franky never touched you and that he never beat you or your siblings. What about the bruises on Junior and Alicia? What about your bruises?" the investigator asked, but I already had rehearsed the answers in my mind long before he directed the questions to me.

"We fight a lot. We hit each other, you know as siblings do; just sibling rivalry, Mr. Walton; we play rough," I answered and, with superficial indifference, looked away from his penetrating eyes.

"Just a rivalry, uh-huh." He repeated my words, holding his gaze on me.

"That's right. Just sibling rivalry." I stood firm under the permeating beams of his studying eyes. The people who had filled the office left, and I found myself again seated in front of the bearded man and the woman in the flowery dress. For a long time, they continued asking questions. The pressure on me became unbearable. They repeatedly returned to the same questions and asked about the same things. I became confused. I wanted out.

"I want Victoria...," I said, exhausted by their unceasing bombardment of questions. "I want Victoria...," I repeated and vowed to speak no more.

The woman in the flowery dress trotted on her high heels out of the room, and I could hear her talking to someone, asking,

"Who is Victoria? Bella is very distressed and wants to see Victoria. Is that somebody from her family? Is Victoria here? Who is Victoria?" she asked some people I could not see.

"Victoria is her social worker, not a family. And she is not here. The foster mother brought Bella to the interview this morning." I heard somebody responding.

"A social worker? The child wants her social worker?" The heels of the woman in the flowery dress trotted back into the room. "They usually want their mothers, not their social workers," I heard her mumbling to herself.

"Mija," the woman approached me and put her arms on my shoulders, "we can call Victoria, and you can talk with her on the phone, but she is not here, sweetie. Maybe we can call her and ask her to see you at the foster home. Do you want that?"

"Yes," I nodded and took some Kleenex tissues she had offered me. I wiped away sweat, not tears. What did she think? Doesn't she know that I can't cry? Doesn't she know that I was dry inside and out? Those drops of sweat rolling down my temples betrayed my fears, not my weakness.

On the way back, I sat in the back seat of the car and thought of Alicia and Junior. I was sure they would be glad to hear that I kept my word and didn't betray them. I denied everything that I had initially told the school about Franky. I felt good about the ground I thought I had conquered for Alicia and Junior. They could go back with Franky and cry no more. The bearded man and the woman in a flowery dress seemed to believe me. Did they? I wondered.

Task: Describe your emotions when reading the story of Alma Bella.

_____
_____
_____
_____
_____
_____

Note: At this point in the healing process, you should have experienced a degree of liberation from pain and oppression. The story of Alma Bella serves as a personal test to assess your recovery through a simple assignment: To generate a response of compassion and empathy. The presence of these emotions indicates a satisfactory level of healing and a spirit that is awakened to the pain of others, responding with genuine empathy. This fulfills one of the objectives of *EHAD with GOD* stated in session one.

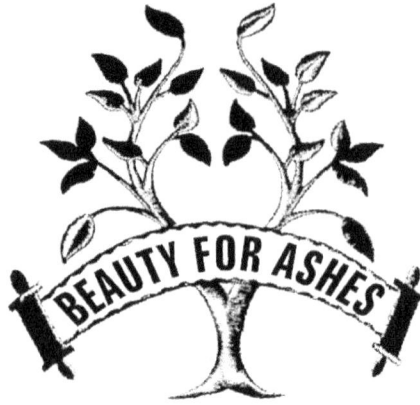

SESSION TEN

THE ARMOR OF GOD

The Enemy

There is a constant spiritual battle going on in the spiritual realm. The accuser, Satan, brings accusations against the believers before God day and night (Revelation 12:10). Our mistakes are his condemnations. When a spiritual law is broken, it allows the enemy to take a "foothold" in the person's heart (Ephesians 4:27). It lodges itself in the human mind and psyche and becomes an intrinsic part of the person's character, bringing destruction. Under these circumstances, the breastplate of righteousness and the shield of faith (Ephesians 6) are no longer impenetrable; the believer is exposed to the flaming arrows of the enemy. Awareness of this spiritual dynamic is a must.

The Earth is the dimension to which Satan was cast down, dragging with himself third of the stars of heaven (angels) (Revelation 12:4). Jesus saw Satan fall like lightning from heaven to earth (Luke 10:18). Satan is the ruler of the kingdom of the air, the spirit who is now at work in those who are disobedient

(Ephesians 2:2). Jesus referred to Satan as "a liar and the father of lies" and a "murderer" (John 8:44), "the prince of this world" (John 12:31), "the enemy" (Matthew 13:39), "the evil one" (Matthew 13:38).

Satan and his demonic hordes are real spiritual entities. Their mission is clear: To entice and deceive humans away from God and drag them down into eternity in hell. God is love; Satan is hate. These fallen forces existed on earth before the creation (Genesis 1). The serpent was already in the Garden of Eden. The Apostle John referred to Satan as the "great dragon" and the "serpent of old" (Revelation 12:9), identifying him as the same entity from the Garden of Eden (Genesis 3).

> The great dragon was thrown down—the ancient serpent
> called the Devil, or Satan, who leads the whole world astray.
> He was hurled to the earth and his angels with him.
> (Revelation 12:9)

The Pharisees accused Jesus of casting out the demons by Beelzebub, Satan himself (Matthew 12:22-32). The Israelites of that epoch had a worldview that offered only two options: The alternative to the power of God was to bow down to the power of Satan (Beelzebub). There was no non-theistic option. The Bible doesn't argue about the existence of God, Satan, angelic, or evil/demonic spirits. The Bible does not speak metaphorically of them and has not changed the understanding of their nature, origin, involvement in human history, or their final destiny. However, Americans' views on the spiritual realm have changed drastically, especially in the last twenty years. A Gallup study in 2023 found that Americans' beliefs regarding God, angels, heaven, hell, and the Devil have fallen by double digits since 2001.

The majority of Americans still believe in the existence of each entity, ranging from a high of 74% believing in God to lows of 59% for hell and 58% for the Devil. Nevertheless, when these indicators were compared with results from 2001, the drop was a staggering two digits. Belief in God and heaven was down the most, with 16 points each, while belief in hell has fallen 12 points, and the Devil and angels are down 10 points each (Figure 2). The results clearly attest to what Jesus referred to as the generation of Noah (Matthew 24:37-39).

> As it was in the days of Noah, so it will be at the coming of the Son of Man. (Matthew 24:37)

Figure 2. Americans' Belief 2001-2023[25]

Americans' Belief in Five Spiritual Entities, 2001-2023

For each of the following items I am going to read you, please tell me whether it is something you believe in, something you're not sure about, or something you don't believe in.

% Believe in

— God — Heaven ···· Angels – – Hell – – The devil

100

90
83
80
79
71
68
60

40
2001 2003 2005 2007 2009 2011 2013 2015 2017 2019 2021 2023

74
69
67
59
58

GALLUP

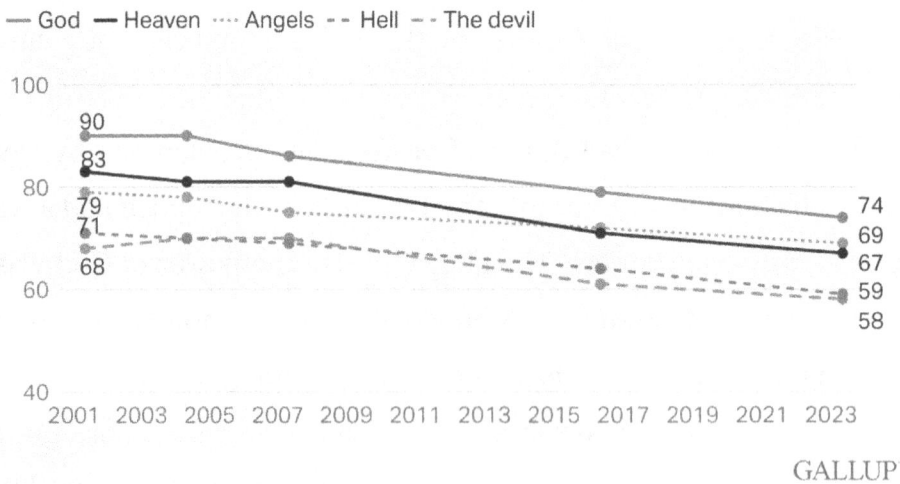

Another study, at the Cultural Research Center at Arizona Christian University, compared the Americans' biblical worldview before (2020) and after (2023) the pandemic[26]. The study confirmed the drastic downward trajectory identified in Gallup polls. The researchers defined three categories of people: Integrated Disciples (strong believers with a biblical worldview), Emergent Followers (nominal Christians), and World Citizens (individuals with

25 Brenan, M. (2023). Belief in Five Spiritual Entities Edges Down to New Lows. Gallup, Washington DC.

26 https://www.arizonachristian.edu/wp-content/uploads/2023/02/CRC_AWVI2023_Release1.pdf

a secular worldview). The first two groups registered 2% and 11% drops in their post-pandemic worldview indicators compared to their values before the pandemic. In contrast, the third secular group registered a 13% increase (see Table 3).

Table 3. Shift in Americans' Biblical Worldview[27]

Groups/Change in %	2020	2023
Integrated Disciples	6	4
Emergent Followers	25	14
World Citizen	69	82

Figure 3. Shift in Americans' Pre- and Postpandemic Worldviews[28]

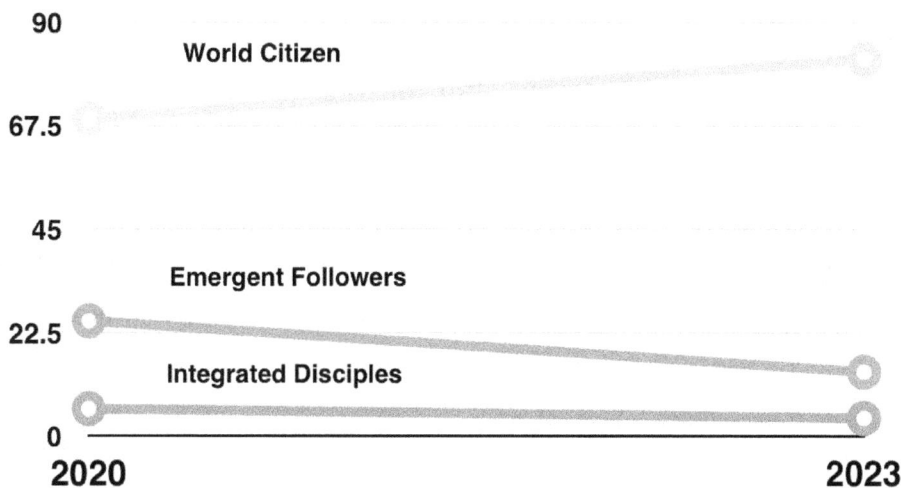

---

[27] Source: American Worldview Inventory, conducted in 2020 and 2023, by the Cultural Research Center at Arizona Christian University. Each study is based on a national sample of 2,000 adults, interviewed by telephone and online in January.

[28] Figure 3 is a visual display of Table 2 on the "Shift in Americans' Biblical Worldview."

The conclusion is obvious: Americans' worldviews have shifted towards secular views, with a significant drop among the believers (Figure 3). While the believers' worldview shifted away from the foundations of the biblical truth, the number of individuals with secular worldviews expanded.

For further reference on heaven and hell, angels and demons, refer to the teaching of John Ramirez[29], a former satanic priest, now an evangelical pastor[30]. He has seen the "other side" of the spiritual realm and attested to the goals, objectives, and strategies of the Devil to take humankind down to hell with him[31].

The disciples asked Jesus about the signs of the last days.

> "Tell us," they said, "when will this happen, and what will be the sign of your coming and of the end of the age?" Jesus answered: "Watch out that no one deceives you." (Matthew 24:3b-4)

Deception is the sign of the last days. Even the elect are targeted for deception (Matthew 24:11,24). Deception is only possible when spiritual slumber exists, the numbing of the heart. Jesus instructed us to be like the wise virgins waiting, with lamps full of oil, prepared for the bridegroom's appearance because no one knows either the day nor the hour in which the Son of Man is coming (Matthew 25:1-13).

We are currently witnessing the era of "the sign of the fig tree" (Matthew 24:32), the signs of the end time. They are prophetically spoken.

1) The return of the Jewish people to their ancestral land. This prophecy was fulfilled on May 14, 1948, with the creation of the state of Israel (Isaiah 11:11; Jeremiah 29:10; Hosea 3:4-5; Amos 9:15; Ezekiel 22:17–22).

---

29 https://johnramirez.org/

30 https://www.youtube.com/watch?v=MQnRJ31c1vU

31 https://www.amazon.com/Exposing-Enemy-Simple-Defeating-Strategies/dp/0768450861?source=ps-sl-shoppingads-lpcontext&ref_=fplfs&psc=1&smid=ATVPDKIKX0DER

2) The Great Apostasy—the falling away, even of the elect (2 Thessalonians 2:3). The data from the research confirms that what we are observing today is indeed the great falling away the Apostle Paul warned about (2 Thessalonians 2:3). This is the end time of human history, ridden with demonic perversion and persecution of the believers.

Jesus warned that, in the last days, because of increased wickedness, the love of many will grow cold (Matthew 24:12). Jesus referred to the divine, agape kind of love, which only believers can attain. The world cannot love with agape love. Apparently, it is God's Church that would grow cold and lack agape love for Him, not the world. In the last days, the Church would fall short of meeting the righteous requirement of the first commandment: To love the Lord God with all mind, soul, and strength. The research data confirms this sad trend.

Apostle Paul described the signs of the last days.

> But mark this: There will be terrible times in the last days. People will be lovers of themselves, lovers of money, boastful, proud, abusive, disobedient to their parents, ungrateful, unholy, without love, unforgiving, slanderous, without self-control, brutal, not lovers of the good, treacherous, rash, conceited, lovers of pleasure rather than lovers of God— having a form of godliness but denying its power. Have nothing to do with such people. (2 Timothy 3:1-5)

We are called to endure even when persecuted.

> In fact, everyone who wants to live a godly life in Christ Jesus will be persecuted, while evil men and impostors will go from bad to worse, deceiving and being deceived. (2 Timothy 3:12-13)

How are we to endure? The believer must attain the Armor of God. The Apostle Paul eloquently described the Armor of God in his letter to the Ephesians.

Finally, be strong in the Lord and in   his mighty power. Put on the full armor of God so that you can take your stand against the devil's schemes. For our struggle is not against flesh and blood, but against the rulers, against the authorities, against the powers of this dark world and against the spiritual forces of evil in the heavenly realms.

Therefore, put on the full armor of God, so that when the day of evil comes, you may be able to stand your ground, and after you have done everything, to stand. Stand firm then, with the belt of truth buckled around your waist, with the breastplate of righteousness in place, and with your feet fitted with the readiness that comes from the gospel of peace. In addition to all this, take up the shield of faith, with which you can extinguish all the flaming arrows of the evil one. Take the helmet of salvation and the sword of the Spirit, which is the word of God.

And pray in the Spirit on all occasions with all kinds of prayers and requests. With this in mind, be alert and always keep on praying for all the saints. (Ephesians 6:10-18)

The images associated with the Armor of God depict a Roman soldier in full battle gear. The description does fit the image of that time, but Apostle Paul didn't derive it from the Romans. In his letter to the Ephesians, he referred to Isaiah 59. Long before the Roman Empire even existed, the Prophet Isaiah described the same image.

> The Lord looked and was displeased that there was no justice. He saw that there was no one, he was appalled that there was no one to intervene; so his own arm achieved salvation for him, and his own righteousness sustained him. He put on righteousness as his breastplate, and the helmet of salvation on his head; he put on the garments of vengeance and wrapped himself in zeal as in a cloak. (Isaiah 59:15-17)

Notice that, in his description, Apostle Paul skipped the elements of "the cloak of zeal" as part of God's "garments of vengeance." Instead, we are fitted with a garment of peace—the readiness that comes from the gospel of peace. The omission is intentional. It is not the function of God's warrior to engage in vengeance; it is God to avenge. Instead, Apostle Paul advises,

> Do not take revenge, my friends, but leave room for God's wrath, for it is written: 'It is mine to avenge; I will repay' says the Lord. (Romans 12:19, Deuteronomy 32:35)

Apostle Paul further encouraged believers,

> Do not repay anyone evil for evil. Be careful to do what is right in the eyes of everyone. If it is possible, as far as it depends on you, live at peace with everyone. (Romans 12:17,18)

Further, quoting Proverbs 25, Apostle Paul directs the believers,

> If your enemy is hungry, feed him; if he is thirsty, give him something to drink. In doing this, you will heap burning coals on his head. (Proverbs 25:21,22)

Zeal is a desirable characteristic of a believer. We are encouraged to be fervent, passionate, and intense for God's cause through devotion, service, and righteousness. In contrast, Isaiah 59 describes the wrath of God, who is wrapped in a cloak as a zeal to repay the evil its due (Isaiah 59:18,19). Jesus displayed this zeal when He drove the money changers out of the Temple because they profaned the House of God, turning it into a marketplace (Matthew 21:12-13; Mark 11:15-18). This kind of righteous indignation becomes part of the believers' character when they are transformed in the image of Christ.

Our battles against evil are still God's battles. Our Armor of God is He Himself living in us. Our prayers are the weapons doing exactly what Isaiah 59 described, driving God to avenge our enemies.

How Do I Acquire the Armor of God?

If you have diligently completed the five steps of the EHAD prayer (page 13) you have already attained the Armor of God. First, you have confessed, rejected, and crucified the old practices of the flesh (discussed at length in sessions one through five). You removed Satan's foothold, refusing him the right to deceive and harass you. You have demolished the stronghold of darkness that held your life hostage to destruction. You have freed yourself from evil dominion and spiritual oppression. You have washed in the blood of Jesus (session four). Your life is now cleansed, purified, and sanctified. You have closed all legal entry of the enemy through any generational line (session eight). At last, you have filled your "house" with the Spirit of the living God, making agape love an inherent part of your godly character (session 9). This is the scriptural understanding of self-deliverance. You have consecrated and sanctified yourself.

In obedience to God's Word, you stepped in faith and fought for your freedom against spiritual dominion and oppression. You acquired the full Armor of God. Your "breastplate of righteousness" is Christ's righteousness in you, imparted as a permanent character trait. Because Christ lives in you, it is not your righteousness and holiness but His righteousness and holiness manifesting in your life now. The "shield of faith" is your new level of awareness and personal conviction of the truthfulness of the Bible and Christ as your Lord, God, and Savior. Your "helmet of salvation" is the stamp of the Holy Spirit with whom you are sealed for eternity (Ephesians 1:13). Your "belt of truth" is your testimony to what Christ has done for you. The greatest of all these blessings is the impartation of agape love. Apostle Paul elevates agape love as the essential attribute of the Armor of God. It is the most refined weapon in the arsenal of the Armor of God, which believers must attain.

> But since we belong to the day, let us be self-controlled, putting on faith and love [agape] as a breastplate and the hope of salvation as a helmet. (1 Thessalonians 5:8)

Lack of agape love is a weakness in the Armor of God. Jesus loves us with agape love, and we must reciprocate with agape love also. This agape love can be attained only through obedience to His commandments (John 14:15,23-24). Jesus' words, "If you love me," refer to the divine agape love. To keep the commandments, the believer must attain agape love to reciprocate Jesus' love. And the believer must obey the commandments to achieve agape love. No, it is not a paradoxical situation of contradictory rules. The obedience to His commandments is the prerequisite, not the other way around.

At this point, you have acquired all the above attributes of the Armor of God. Wielding the "sword of the Spirit" threatens the kingdom of darkness and pushes wickedness away. You are to trample on snakes and scorpions with no fear of harm (Luke 10:19). You are given the power and the authority to do "violence" to the kingdom of darkness just by speaking the Word of God, thus establishing God's will on earth as it is in heaven (Matthew 6:10). The prayer of a righteous person is powerful and effective (James 5:16). You have become more and more like Christ because you have sanctified your life. You are now EHAD with Christ. Your Armor of God is Christ in you, the hope of glory (Colossians 1:27).

Question: How do I put on the full Armor of God? How do I practically put on the breastplate of righteousness? Refer to page 5, Session 1, for a comparison of your answer. How did your understanding change? Discuss your findings.

_____
_____
_____
_____
_____
_____
_____
_____
_____

Royal Priesthood

In your journey of becoming EHAD with GOD, you have come to a high place on the narrow road, a spiritually elevated place where you are called to partake in the duties of a royal priesthood. This is the place for which King David prayed in the anguish of his heart, "Lead me to the rock that is higher than I" (Psalms 61:2). May this also be our prayer of ascent, may his longing be our longing as we wait for the royal and priestly heritage of those who fear God's name. Apostle Peter calls the believers a royal priesthood.

> But you are a chosen people, a royal priesthood, a holy nation, God's special possession, that you may declare the praises of him who called you out of darkness into his wonderful light. (1 Peter 2:9)

From a biblical theology perspective, "royalty" and "priesthood" are never to be linked together. The Law strictly delineated the office of the king and the office of the priest. It was prohibited and punishable by death if a king was to engage in priestly duties and vice versa. The prophet Samuel rebuked King Saul for the burnt offering he officiated at Gilgal, assuming the duties of the priest. The offense was so great that the Kingdom was taken away from Saul and given to one, "the Lord has sought for Himself a man after His own heart"(1 Samual 13:13,14).

Aaron's two sons, Nadab and Abihu, died after offering unauthorized, "foreign fire" to God. They acted in violation of God's instructions and were consumed by the flames (Leviticus 10). The Book of Numbers outlines the duties of the Kohathites, a family within the Levite tribe. They were charged with transporting the holy objects of the Tabernacle when the camp was ready to move. All furnishings had to be covered by the priests, Aaron and his sons. If Kohathies touched any of the holy furnishings, they would die (Numbers 4:15). Even well-meaning priests who exceeded their duties, coming into contact with a holy object, were punished by death. And yet, Apostle Peter is calling the believers "royal priesthood." What had transpired on the Cross of Jesus that the believers are now endowed with these two offices? Where does this new identity come from? How is the believer to perform these new, simultaneously royal and priestly duties without the threat of death?

The unity of the offices of the king and the priest is not a New Testament concept. The Old Testament scripture prophesied the coming of a divine figure who would unite both offices. Jesus fulfilled the prophecy. The Cross attributed to Him the titles King and High Priest. What is the spiritual mechanism through which the believers also acquire the title "royal priesthood?"

The Office of the Priest

The office of the priesthood was set by the Law of Moses. Before the Law, the heads of the families acted as priests. Job purified his children, sacrificing for them (Job 1:5). Noah (Genesis 8:20), Abraham (Genesis 12:7,8; 13:18), Isaac (Genesis 26:25), Jacob (Genesis 31:54; 35:1-4), they all sacrificed animals to atone for their families. They all built elaborate altars, a place with a special spiritual significance in their encampments, creating sacred spaces in their journeys. The altar was not only a memorial in honor of God, a place of worship, and remembrance of God's faithfulness, but a place of sacrifice, a slaughterhouse, where the life of an animal was exchanged for the life of a human. The altar is an ugly, bloody, smelly, insect-infested place, a butcher shop, a death-bound place—a graphic depiction of the deadly consequences of sin. At the same time, the sacrifice offered was considered holy, and everything it touched, its flesh or blood, was considered consecrated and made holy also (Leviticus 6:27). The sacrifice became holy because the altar was holy. Moses received special instructions on how to consecrate the altar of the Tabernacle. It required a seven-day ritual involving anointing with oil and the application of the sacrificial blood of a bull and a ram (Exodus 29). Their blood was sprinkled on the horns and the base of the altar, thus making it holy. Only after its consecration, the altar became holy. The holiness was transferred through contact; its holiness was "contagious." Today, when an altar call is given, be reminded of the grotesque sight of the Cross of Jesus, where a spiritual transaction happened: The profane became holy through the holiness of our Lord. It was God's will that "we have been made holy through the sacrifice of the body of Jesus Christ once for all" (Hebrews 10:10).

The Law of Moses introduced to the Israelites new ways of communicating with God, setting strict boundaries and expectations for a new sacrificial system. The place of meeting was the Tabernacle, also called the Tent of the Meeting, and the conditions for meeting were codified in the duties of specially appointed offices. Aaron and his descendants were to act as priests (Exodus 29:44; 30:30; Numbers 3:10), and the tribe of Levi was called to help in the care of the structure and the functions of the Tabernacle (Numbers 1:50,51,53). The rest of the people were prohibited from participating or coming close to the altar. They were mere silent observers. At the same time, they were the beneficiaries of the arrangements made.

The priests and the Levites were the intercessors between God and the people. To function as such, they had to be consecrated into the service and maintain the sanctity of their spiritual status. They had to be continuously holy to the Lord. If the status is lost, the reconsecration of the high priest required the ashes of a red heifer (Numbers 19:1-2), a ceremony of "water of separation" to cleanse those who have become ritually unclean. This is a challenging task for Israel today. If a Third Temple practice is to be established, it requires a legitimately consecrated high priest. According to the Jewish tradition, since Aaron, there have been only nine red heifers sacrificed for the consecration of the high priests. As of today, out of the five unblemished heifers transported to Israel from Texas in September 2022,[32] only two are currently considered eligible. They continue to be monitored to ensure their eligibility according to Old Testament standards.

Along with all required priestly attire (Exodus 28), God also ordered,

---

[32] https://ffoz.org/messiah/articles/did-we-just-sacrifice-a-red-heifer-for-real

Make a plate of pure gold and engrave on it as on a seal: **holy to the Lord**. Fasten a blue cord to it to attach it to the turban; it is to be on the front of the turban. It will be on Aaron's forehead, and he will bear the guilt involved in the sacred gifts the Israelites consecrate, whatever their gifts may be. It will be on Aaron's forehead continually so that they will be acceptable to the Lord. (Exodus 28: 36,38)

The priest had to be holy. He was the direct access to God for the common person. When the priests acted wickedly, the dereliction of their duty became a stench in God's nostrils (Isaiah 65:5; Amos 4:10). Their defilement defiled the temple, and the sacrifices they offered were not acceptable to God (Proverbs 15:8; Psalms 40:6-8; Isaiah 1:11-31; Jeremiah 7:21-23). The offense resulted in God departing from the temple (Ezekiel 10:18), and the Babylonian exile followed.

Old Testament history informs the New Testament believer in all spiritual matters related to the priesthood. The New Covenant came with a new Temple structure. **First**, Jesus removed the barrier between God and the common worshiper. The symbolic tear of the Temple's curtain, upon Jesus' death, separating the Holy of Holies, also tore the separation of God and people (Matthew 27:51). Everyone could now approach God. **Second**, the day of Pentecost (Acts 2) created a new spiritual entity, a body of believers, a body of Christ that became the new Temple. To partake in Temple service, the believers must attain and maintain the same holiness as required for the ancient Aaronic priests. Otherwise, just like in the Old Testament story, God will not be present. Apostle Paul writes,

Don't you know that you yourselves are God's temple and that God's Spirit dwells in your midst? (1 Corinthians 3:16)

While the Temple structures changed, the functions of the priests didn't. The access to God was now dependent upon the consecration of each believer. Prophetically, Isaiah 61 described this new reality.

> And you will be called priests of the Lord, you will be named ministers of our God. (Isaiah 61:6)

This statement precedes the event, also prophesied in the same Scripture, which Jesus read, when He first identified Himself as the anointed one who came to proclaim the good news to the poor (Isaiah 61:1). The entire text of Isaiah 61:1-5 describes the duties of a high priest, duties Jesus assumed after His sacrifice on the Cross. According to the prophecy, the believers in Jesus are also priests and ministers (Isaiah 61:6).

The Apostle John further affirmed this spiritual appointment. He goes even further

> To him who loves us and has freed us from our sins by his blood, and has made us to be a kingdom and priests to serve his God and Father—to him be glory and power for ever and ever! Amen. (Revelation 1:6)

The call to be priests of the Lord is the believers' destiny. Along with this honor comes the responsibility to acquire and maintain the same Old Testament criteria of holiness. The Lord had not waived the requirements for purity. Jesus repeatedly said,

> Be perfect, therefore, as your heavenly Father is perfect. (Matthew 5:48).

Apostle Peter, quoting the Old Testament (Leviticus 11:44,45; 19:2), echoed the command,

> But just as he who called you is holy, so be holy in all you do; for it is written: "Be holy, because I am holy." (1 Peter 1:15,16)

How do believers achieve and maintain the status of holiness acceptable to the Lord? The duty of the Old Testament priests was to offer sacrifice as an act of worship, atoning for sins, expressing gratitude, showing devotion, and restoring a right relationship with God for themselves and on behalf of the people. Similarly, Apostle Paul calls the believers to offer themselves as a living sacrifice on the altar of Jesus, which is the Cross, as true and proper worship.

> Therefore, I urge you, brothers and sisters, in view of God's mercy, to offer your bodies as a living sacrifice, holy and pleasing to God—this is your true and proper worship. (Romans 12:1)

This is the spiritual act of offering oneself as a burnt offering, a pleasing aroma to the Lord (Leviticus 1:9). Burning the old nature on the altar of God is equivalent to "take your cross daily" (Luke 9:23). It is a spiritual act of spiritually crucifying the old self with Christ (Galatians 2:20), and putting to death whatever belongs to the earthly nature (Colossians 3:5). It is an act of faith to move from death to life.

> For if you live according to the flesh, you will die; but if by the Spirit you put to death the misdeeds of the body, you will live. (Romans 8:13)

When we sacrifice the old self on the altar of Christ, the Cross, we perform a priestly duty. We are consecrated and sanctified; everything that the holy altar of Christ touches becomes holy. No red heifer is needed; the Cross and the blood of Christ accomplished the task. We have been made holy through the sacrifice of the body of Jesus Christ once for all (Hebrews 10:10). The holiness is a prerequisite for the power and the authority of Christ to be vested in us (Matthew 10:1; Luke 10:19). We became eligible to serve as priests to others, bringing them to the altar of Christ, leading them to gain the same spiritual benefit. This is Jesus' command known as the Great Commission.

> All authority in heaven and on earth has been given to me. Therefore, go and make disciples of all nations, baptizing them in the name of the Father and of the Son and of the Holy Spirit, and teaching them to obey everything I have

commanded you. And surely I am with you always, to the
very end of the age. (Matthew 28:16-20)

Discipleship is the duty of all believers. New followers are to move from spiritual milk to a solid food spiritual diet quickly, so they can be equipped for the work in the Kingdom of God (Ephesians 4:11, 12). If left by themselves, the new believers are easy prey for the enemy. The parable of the sower illustrates the sad reality. If not equipped, the new believers might fall in those 75% who would not produce a crop, a hundred, sixty, or thirty times what was sown (Matthew 13). The consequence is eternal separation from God. Jesus further solidifies this understanding, saying, "The tree that doesn't produce fruit is cut down and thrown into the fire" (Matthew 7:19; Matthew 21:19). A branch that doesn't bear fruit is thrown away and withers; such branches are picked up, thrown into the fire and burned (John 15:6). The teaching is clear: If we don't take our duties seriously, serving as priests, we are just like the Old Testament spectators, but in our situation, spectators without the eternal destiny with God. Through the victory of Christ on the cross, we are now judicially positioned, in prayer, just like the ancient priests, to evoke changes in the spiritual and natural realms.

Question: Have you been fruitful and multiplied, producing a crop, a hundred, sixty, or thirty times what was sown?

_____
_____
_____
_____
_____
_____
_____
_____
_____
_____
_____

The Office of the King

Professor Daniel Boyarin from the University of California, Berkeley, has contributed to understanding the Jewish roots of the New Testament. His work, *The Jewish Gospels*[33], brings clarity to two of Jesus' titles, Son of God and Son of Man. The prevailing understanding within the body of believers is that the first denotes Jesus' divinity and the second, his humanity. This understanding, however, differs from the understanding of the first-century Jewish believers.

Jesus—the Son of God

Apostle Mark introduced Jesus as the "Son of God" (Mark 1:1). According to Scripture, all kings of Israel from the Davidic line are called "sons of God." Apostle Mark makes the claim that Jesus is the prophesied new King of Israel who comes from the Davidic dynasty. He established Jesus' royal line of succession to the throne of King David. Psalm 2 is the official coronation liturgy of an Israelite king and includes this understanding of Father/son relationship.

> I have installed my king on Zion, my holy mountain. I will proclaim the Lord's decree: He said to me, 'You are my **son;** today I have become your **father.**' (Psalms 2:6,7)

Further, all kings of Israel are also called messiahs, meaning the anointed one. Upon their divine election, they were literary anointed with oil. The Prophet Samuel took a vial of oil and poured it upon Saul's head, declaring him "prince" over God's inheritance (1 Samuel 10:1). Other Israelite kings have also been anointed with oil on their accession to the kingship, including David (1 Samuel 16:3), Solomon (1 Kings 1:34), Jehu (1 Kings 19:16), Joash (2 Kings 11:12), and Jehoahaz (2 Kings 23:30). The kings were not divine, but they were elevated by God, endowed with special wisdom, protection, and favor. This was valid for all Israel's kings, and therefore, they are referred to in the Hebrew Bible as the Anointed of God or the Messiahs of God.

---

33 Boyarin, D. (2012) The Jewish Gospels: The Story of the Jewish Christ. The New Press, New York

The title "Son of God" refers to a Davidic king, not a divine figure. God, through the Prophet Nathan, established the throne of King David forever. The recorded promise for King Solomon describes a unique human/divine relationship, "I will be his **father**, and he will be my **son**"(2 Samuel 7:14; 1 Chronicles 28:6). Yet, an Israelite king, anointed and "adopted" by God, was never considered divine.

Jesus is called the Branch, a shoot from the stump of Jesse, King David's father. The prophecies highlight His Davidic and royal ancestry (Isaiah 11:1, Jeremiah 23:5), thus validating His title as the "Son of God."

The title "Son of God" also refers to Jesus' divine origin as the Son of the Father in heaven. While His human ancestry traces back to King David, His divine conception positions Him as the Son of God, the Father. For the first century, Jewish eyewitnesses, Jesus was the "Son of God," the long-awaited divine Messiah from the ancestral line of David.

Interestingly, the spiritual entities, angels and demons, knew who Jesus was. The angel Gabriel called Him "Son of the Most High" and "Son of God" (Luke 1:32,35). The demon possessed from the region of the Gerasenes called Him "Son of God" (Luke 8:26-39; Mark 5:1-20). The impure spirit that came out of a man called Him "Holy One of God." In the Gospels, humans and spiritual beings validated Jesus as the "Son of God."

The Babylonian exile severed the Davidic line of succession. At the time of Jesus, the Jews were still awaiting the absent king to be revealed. When Apostle Mark called Jesus the Son of God, he was asserting this understanding, establishing the prophetic connection of Jesus as the anointed King, the Messiah, the Anointed One from the line of King David. The Gospels of Matthew and Luke also established Jesus' succession to the Davidic throne (Matthew 1; Luke 3:23-38), calling Him "the son of God from the line of Adam" (Luke 3:38) and Christ, the Anointed One (Matthew 1:16). Both references position Jesus as the long-awaited absent King of the Jews from the Davidic line.

Jesus—the Son of Man

Jesus repeatedly referred to Himself as the "Son of Man" (Mark 2:10; 9:9; Matthew 25:31-46; Luke 19:10; 9:56; 19:10). In the Gospel of John alone, Jesus called Himself the "Son of Man" twelve times (1:51; 3:13, 14; 5:27; 6:27, 53, 62; 8:28; 9:35; 12:23; 12:34; 13:31). This is the second title associates with Jesus. Neither His followers nor the Pharisees asked why Jesus called Himself the Son of Man, because they all knew the Scripture which described one like a Son of Man, a divine figure introduced by the Prophet Daniel (Daniel 7:13). The Israelites of Jesus' time were very familiar with the meaning of the title. Just as they were awaiting the earthly king from the line of David, the Son of God, they also awaited the divine figure of the Son of Man to be revealed. According to the Prophet Daniel's description, the Son of Man is both human and divine. The Jews were very well informed of the prophecy.

> In my vision at night, I looked, and there before me was one like a son of man, coming with the clouds of heaven. He approached the Ancient of Days and was led into his presence. He was given authority, glory, and sovereign power; all nations and peoples of every language worshiped him. His dominion is an everlasting dominion that will not pass away, and his kingdom is one that will never be destroyed. (Daniel 7:13,14)

"Coming on the clouds" is an expression and a biblical association of divinity and clouds. It is a statement that the man Daniel saw in his vision had a divine nature. Daniel was given an earth-shattering vision of prophetic revelation. It was a history-changing event. He received the vision of the future divine Messiah. At the time of the vision, Daniel didn't know the enormity of the event. A new theological concept was born; a new progressive revelation from the God of Israel was given. This is a new theological postulation of a human appearing as a deity to whom the title of Son of Man is given. The concept is a major milestone in Judaism from which the messianic theology is derived.

The attributes of the Son of Man, as the Prophet Daniel described them, are: He is human but also divine, comes in the clouds, occupies the throne, next to God, and is given dominion on earth, sovereignty over the entire world, and Gentiles and Jews will one day be His subjects. Daniel described what he saw, but he didn't know what it meant, even when one of the holy servants of God explained it to him. The Apostles, however, saw these attributes in Jesus and identified him as the divine figure of the Son of Man from Daniel's vision. The apostles recognized the fulfillment of Daniel's prophecy.

Jesus didn't coin the term Son of Man. This was a 500-year-old term within Judaism; it was widely known. According to Professor Boyarin[34], Jesus embodies the fulfillment of a rather common expectation of a divine Messiah. Long prior to His coming, the Babylonian Talmud, the rabbinic scholars, had built the understanding of the mysterious Son of Man of Daniel's vision. Many references to Christ, the Anointed One, also come from terminology used by the Essenes of Qumran (Dead Sea Scrolls). If Jesus were inventing new concepts or theology, people of His time would not have understood Him. When Jesus arrived, there was a widespread expectation of a divine Messiah. The New Testament writers identified Jesus as the divine Messiah whom the Jewish people expected.

The Apostle John narrates an interesting exchange between Jesus and common Jewish fishermen who were very familiar with Daniel's Son of Man and the Davidic Son of God concepts. Philip found Nathanael and told him,

> We have found the one Moses wrote about in the Law, and about whom the prophets also wrote—Jesus of Nazareth, the son of Joseph. (John 1:44-48)

After a short exchange, Nathaniel, the unschooled fisherman, identified Jesus as the Son of God, the king of Israel.

---

34 Boyarin, D. (2012) The Jewish Gospels: The Story of the Jewish Christ. The New Press, New York, p. 33

Then Nathanael declared, "Rabbi, you are the **Son of God**; you are the **king of Israel**."(John 1:44-49)

Jesus didn't deny his acknowledgment but added a new revelation, introducing Himself as the Son of Man,

"Very truly I tell you, you will see heaven open, and the angels of God ascending and descending on the **Son of Man.**" (John 1:51)

By claiming the title, the Son of Man, Jesus further revealed His identity. Jesus didn't introduce a new concept. The fishermen were not confused because they knew the prophecies Philip referred to (John 1:45). The title belonged only to the divine Messiah. Their enthusiasm is transparent throughout the narrative. They didn't follow a political figure but a heavenly one. Nathaniel's quick recognition of Jesus confirms this fact. Jesus always said that He was the One to whom the prophets and the Torah had been pointing and whom Daniel had spoken of.

To solidify his claim, in His conversation with Nathaniel, Jesus referenced Jacob's dream of a ladder to heaven. He was most likely alluding to Himself as the gate to heaven, the house of God (Genesis 28:10-17), a place where God and humans connect. And He was the representative of both God and humanity. He affirmed His authority over this divine position, saying, "I am the way and the truth and the life. No one comes to the Father except through me" (John 14:6). The fishermen understood the claim because they knew the Scripture.

Another confirmation of the above-stated fact can be witnessed during the gathering of chief priests and the whole Sanhedrin, who were looking for evidence against Jesus so that they could put him to death (Mark 14:55-64).

The high priest asked him, "Are you the Messiah, the Son of the Blessed One?" "I am," said Jesus. "And you will see the Son of Man sitting at the right hand of the Mighty One and coming on the clouds of heaven." (Mark 14:61-62)

The High Priest asked two critical questions: "Are you the Messiah?" and "Are you the Son of God?" The questions were intended to establish whether Jesus was the anointed, new kingly leader of the Jews from the Davidic dynasty. This is a strictly political question to which Jesus responded, "I am". The high priest remained composed, accepting the claim as fact. His reaction, however, went ballistic at Jesus' second claim as the Son of Man. He tore his clothes and called the claim a blasphemy. The title Son of God was not offensive or punishable, but the title Son of Man was a death sentence because it claimed that Jesus was God, a blasphemy. The irony could not be more striking: The elite who studied the Scripture didn't recognize Him; the poor fishermen who were taught by the elite did. Jesus addressed this sad reality, saying,

> I praise you, Father, Lord of heaven and earth, because you
> have hidden these things from the wise and learned, and
> revealed them to little children. (Matthew 11:25)

The Scripture spoke prophetically of Jesus as the coming divine King. And yet, the scholars of His time missed the message.

> For to us a child is born, to us a son is given, and the
> government will be on his shoulders. And he will be called
> Wonderful Counselor, Mighty God,
> Everlasting Father, Prince of Peace.
> ...He will reign on David's throne and over his kingdom,
> establishing and upholding it with justice and
> righteousness from that time on and forever. (Isaiah 9:6,7)

Jesus Himself confirmed his divine kingship a second time when questioned by Pontius Pilate.

> My kingdom is not of this world. If it were, my servants
> would fight to prevent my arrest by the Jewish leaders. But
> now my kingdom is from another place. (John 18:36)

Apostle Paul, referring to the above exchange between Jesus and Pontius Pilate, when writing to Timothy, called Jesus King of kings and Lord of lords— divine titles.

> In the sight of God, who gives life to everything, and of Christ Jesus, who while testifying before Pontius Pilate made the good confession, I charge you to keep this command without spot or blame until the appearing of our Lord Jesus Christ, which God will bring about in his own time—God, the blessed and only Ruler, the **King of kings and Lord of lords**. (1 Timothy 6:13-15)

Royalty to the believers is attributed via adoption into the family of God. Those who "receive him, who believed in his name, he gave the right to become children of God" (John 1:12). The new identity transformed the believers from "strangers and aliens" into "members of the household of God" (Ephesians 2:19). Because of the work of the Spirit, who resurrected the spirits of the believers upon confession of faith (John 3:16), they are now considered legally adopted by the living God. The Apostle Paul refers to this spiritual adoption, using the specific legal Greek terminology "adoption to sonship." This is the mechanism that gives full legal standing to an adopted male heir in Roman culture.

> The Spirit you received does not make you slaves, so that you live in fear again; rather, the Spirit you received brought about your adoption to sonship. And by him we cry, "Abba, Father." (Romans 8:15)

The office of the King and the Priest—The Royal Priesthood

The Scripture foretold of a Messiah who is simultaneously king and priest (Psalms 110:4; Zachariah 6:13). King David prophesied of another person who, like Melchizedek, holds the priestly and kingly offices.

> You are a priest forever, in the order of Melchizedek.
>
> (Psalms 110:4)

Melchizedek was a king of Salem and a priest. He met Abraham with bread and wine and blessed him in the name of God Most High. As a sign of recognition and gratitude, Abraham gave him a tenth of everything he owned (Genesis 14:17-20).

In his long discourse, the author of the letter to the Hebrews compares Jesus to Melchizedek. The Law of Moses has designated the priesthood only to the descendants of Aaron and the tribe of Levi. Neither Jesus nor Melchizedek is a descendant of this tribe. Even more, Melchizedek preceded the Law of Moses. The Law and the priesthood, the author argues, were powerless to bring perfection in righteousness. Only Jesus made it possible for humanity to attain holiness, enabling believers to meet the righteous requirements of the Law. This is the main duty of a priest—to serve as a medium, reconciling people with God. Jesus fulfilled the prophecies. He "became priest not on the basis of a regulation as to his ancestry but on the basis of the power of an indestructible life" (Hebrews 7:16). Thus, God changed the old order of things, declaring in an oath, "You are a priest forever! (Psalms 104:4). Because of this oath, Jesus has become the guarantor of a better covenant. And because Jesus lives forever, he has a permanent priesthood. Therefore, he can save those who come to God through him, because he always lives to intercede for them (Hebrews 7:23-25).

The Law appoints as priests men in all their weakness who sin, like Hophni and Phinehas (1 Samuel 2:12-4:11), and thus lead others to sin. They had to sacrifice for their own sin and for the sins of the people. This old order of things was changed through the perfect sacrifice of Jesus. The oath of God appointed Jesus, who has been made perfect forever, holy, blameless, pure, set apart from sinners, exalted above the heavens. This is the new covenant God promised through the Prophet Jeremiah, "

> The time is coming," declares the LORD, "when I will make a new covenant with the house of Israel and with the house of Judah. It will not be like the covenant I made with their forefathers when I took them by the hand to lead them out of Egypt, because they broke my covenant, though I was a husband to them," declares the LORD. "This is the covenant I will make with the house of Israel after that time," declares the LORD. "I will put my law in their minds and write it on their hearts. I will be their God, and they will be my people. No longer will a man teach his neighbor, or a man his brother, saying, 'Know the LORD,' because they will all know me, from the least of them to the greatest," declares the LORD. "For I will forgive their wickedness and will remember their sins no more." (Jeremiah 31:31-34)

Jesus entered the Most Holy Place once and for all by his own blood, thus obtaining eternal redemption. He has appeared once for all at the culmination of the ages to do away with sin by the sacrifice of himself (Hebrews 8:26). He became the high priest of the new order of things prophesied by the Prophet Jeremiah. And the believers are the beneficiaries because His priesthood introduced a "better hope by which believers draw near to God" (Hebrews 7:19).

The Prophet Zachariah also spoke of a coming high priest who is king. He was commanded to make a crown of silver and gold and set it on the head of the high priest, Joshua son of Jozadak, saying,

> Here is the man whose name is the Branch, and he will branch out from his place and build the temple of the Lord. It is he who will build the temple of the Lord, and

> he will be clothed with majesty and will sit and rule on his
> throne. And he will be a priest on his throne. And there will
> be harmony between the two.

Jesus is the "high priest on his throne," prophesied by the Prophet Zachariah. He built the temple of the Lord through the body of believers, of which Apostle Paul speaks as the temple of God in which God's Spirit dwells (1 Corinthians 3:16).

Conclusion

There is no **Royal Priesthood** without acquiring the Armor of God. And for an impenetrable Armor of God, the believers must become priests, ministers to our God (Isaiah 61:6). The *EHAD with GOD* approach for sanctification propels the believers from passive pew observers to active field workers, harvesting for the Kingdom of God (Matthew 9:35-38). A believer who wholeheartedly assumes the duties of the royal priesthood is no longer called a servant of God because he/she has become a friend of God.

> I no longer call you servants, because a servant does not
> know his master's business. Instead, I have called you
> friends, for everything that I learned from my Father, I
> have made known to you. (John 15:15)

Question: How does Jesus call you?

_____
_____
_____
_____
_____
_____
_____
_____
_____

BEWARE!!!

Applying the principles of *EHAD with GOD* radically changes your life, aligning it with the kingdom of God, rejecting the kingdom of darkness. Once you were oppressed and harassed by the enemy, but now you are free from captivity to sin. You have demolished the power of the strongholds over your life. You have broken the cycle of sin and death, and you have chosen life instead. The enemy is not "happy"; he is indeed raging over his "loss." He will throw at you every lie, deception, seduction, and unfortunate event with the only goal to discourage you from living up to what you have already attained, your victory in Christ (Philippians 3:16). There will be doubts planted in your mind that the *EHAD with GOD* biblical approach doesn't work. It is a lie! *EHAD with GOD* is based on spiritual laws that were set at the beginning of time. When applied in faith, they bring fulfillment on earth as it was ordained in heaven. Be aware! There will be attacks, maybe relentless attacks. Be warned: The enemy, the devil, prowls around like a roaring lion looking for someone to devour (1 Peter 5:8).

What shall your response be? Be on your knees in prayer and supplication (Philippians 4:6). Make *EHAD with GOD* way of the cross a daily routine; practice the spiritual disciplines on the narrow road daily. This is your Armor of God. Stay your ground! Submit to God. Resist the devil, and he will flee from you (James 4:7). Deal with the schemes of the Devil the way Jesus did, rebuking the enemy, "Get behind me, Satan!" (Matthew 16:23). Each time you are confronted with a thought or situation, shout the command in your spirit, "Get behind me, Satan!"

This is a war on your eternal life. You must be victorious! The stories of Abigail and Lili illustrate the extent of the harassment the enemy applies to "steal, kill, and destroy" (John 10:10). Spiritual warfare intensifies significantly when believers become determined to destroy the dark power structures over their lives. The daily prayers of *EHAD with GOD* become your permanent Armor of God.

Spiritual Warfare—the Story of Abigail

Late into the evening, the phone rang; no message was left. The second call recorded a desperate cry for help. "Abigail is screaming uncontrollably. She would not go into her room, rolling on the floor, shaking. I don't know what to do. I am scared. Please, help!" The foster mother sounded very worried. Shaking off the initial disorientation caused by the midnight call, Hanna composed herself quickly and called back immediately, "On my way now," she whispered into the receiver, but the echo carried her voice in low humming through the sleepy house. "I should be back before anyone rises in the morning."Hanna thought, looking at the red lights of the clock glaring back at her with 12:30 AM.

Abigail, a nine-year-old girl, was placed in foster care earlier the same day, after a failed adoption. The biological mother's whereabouts were unknown; the biological father was homeless, with a history of substance abuse, unable to visit or care for Abigail. The adoptive family was the second rejection in her nine years of life. Upon placement, she exhibited high anxiety and intense fear, but no one expected the immense degree of depravity this young child carried in her small heart.

It took Hanna some time to calm the child. She sat down on the bare floor, gently stroking Abigail's golden hair. Her voice, low and steady, slowly began to prevail over the child's sobs. Words of assurance and physical affection soon calmed the child. Abigail lifted her fragile frame and unwillingly sat opposite Hanna. A blank stare met Hanna's worried eyes. The sight of the child pierced her heart. Ocean of pain screamed silently at her.

"What is going on, sweety?" Hanna broke the short moment of silence. Abigail shrugged her shoulders, her head tilted away from Hanna, a mute sign of non-cooperation. Hanna's patience and genuine concern, however, soon changed the child's disposition. A few moments later, Abigail spoke through tears; her body still leaning away from Hanna.

"You will not believe me," she said, her voice wavering through spasmodic sobs, "No one believes me." She repeated a bit louder.

"Try me." Responded Hanna. "Tell me what is bothering you, mi amor."

A deep sigh escaped Abigail's hunched chest as she began speaking.

"There is this girl who comes into my room." Abigail posed for a long moment as she turned toward Hanna, anticipating the usual facial expression of ridicule she always got when telling the previous counselors. No one believed her. Why would Hanna believe her? There was no other girl in the home, how could she? Instead of ridicule, though, Abigail met Hanna's encouraging eyes, as her assuring hands reached for hers.

"She comes close to me. She stares at me for a long time, and I am so afraid. I pull my blanket over because the room becomes so cold. I shiver even under the covers. She touches me, and her fingers are so icy cold." A flood of tears poured down Abigail's beautiful face. "I am so scared. No one believes me. The doctor gave me pills, but they didn't help. The girl is still coming every night." The child pulled her legs toward her chest, wrapped her arms tight around them, and hid her wet face, a desperate attempt to bury the memories that caused her to re-experience the horror all over again.

"I believe you," Hanna said, quickly assessing the situation. "The enemy is harassing this poor child", she whispered to herself. A giant wave of indignation swelled within her. "How dare you, Satan, touch this innocent child. Get your hands off her!" Hanna screamed a prayer in her spirit as she held Abigail in her arms, hoping to lessen the child's pain. "Lord Jesus, rebuke the enemy! Cast it away from Abigail! Set her free! I ask you, Jesus, please summon an angelic army to come and crush the forces of darkness!" The prayer warrior in Hanna rose to the occasion, calling on the heavenly power to fight for the life of the innocent. Her genuine compassion had an immediate response—very soon, Abigail's small body molded perfectly into Hanna's embrace.

The time seemed to stop as a wall-to-wall silence expanded its dominance, replacing the commotion of the previous moments. Two enmeshed souls stood divinely connected: One overflowing with prayer for healing, the other receiving the healing; one springing with living water, the other drinking from the same well of life. Eternity entered, the heavenly court was seated, and a royal decree was issued, "Be free! Be healed!" Hanna's arms became the conduit for divine healing.

"Abigail," Hanna was first to interrupt the sweetness of that moment. She lifted the child's chin, her head still buried in her arms. As their eyes met, a new reality became evident: Trust has replaced fear.

"Listen, Abigail, this is what you should do. This is your room, your territory. No one can enter your room without your permission. Next time, when this girl comes, you must stand your ground and tell her to get out."

The child's eyes expanded in the dim light. "I can just tell her to get out?" The child voiced disbelief at the plausibility of the task.

"It is your room, your bed, your life! No one else but you has full command over your territory. Claim it!" Hanna repeated, assuringly. "Put your foot down and tell the girl, 'Get out of my room! In Jesus' name!'" She must obey.

After a few dry runs of practice, what Abigail should say and do, Hanna left the foster home with Abigail neatly tucked in her bed. The next day, Hanna swung by to follow up on the situation. Abigail ran toward Hanna, jumping in excitement, "It worked!" She exclaimed, "The girl left!"

"Tell me more, Abigail, what happened?" Hanna asked.

Abigail put her arms on her hips, stomped the floor, and shouted, "'Get out of my room, in Jesus' name!' This is what I did, and she left! She didn't come back." Abigail's face beamed with determination. She stood her ground and won. The victory fueled her faith, giving her newly found strength. The contrast with the helpless child, the night before, was drastic. In her first spiritual battle, Abigail exercised her right as a believer to call on the authority of Christ against the oppressive power of the enemy. She overcame. Young in years, yet a giant in faith, she triumphed.

If a nine-year-old girl can take authority over her spiritual life, so can any adult with a child-like faith. Just as Jesus said,

> Truly I tell you, unless you change and become like little
> children, you will never enter the kingdom of heaven. You
> must become like a child. (Matthew 18:3)

Abigail won that first battle. As she matures in faith, she must win the war. For the eternal victory over her life, she must acquire the full armor of God, becoming a part of God's royal priesthood. *EHAD with GOD* equips young and old for the task. You, when under attack, remember to shout authoritatively in your spirit, "Get behind me, Satan!"

Spiritual Warfare—the Story of Lili

The sun and the water, hot and cold, were claiming equal dominance over Lili's bodily sensations. Submerged under the rushing streams, she heard the pastor's final statement, "I baptize you in the name of the Father, the Son, and the Holy Spirit." Neither the harsh cold of the water nor the unbearable heat of the air could subdue the joy of this special day. An unknown power of love burst with heavenly peace within. Her spirit soared on wings like an eagle. Delighted in her own transformation, she prayed for more of the same. Soul and body, mind and spirit quietly submitted, willingly relinquishing the reins of her life to Jesus. The contentment of that moment had no equal. Lili just loudly proclaimed from the rooftop (Matthew 10:27) what Jesus did in the quiet of her prayer room (Matthew 6:6), testifying to the world of being born again by the Spirit of the living God.

The transformation began a few months earlier when she enrolled in the *EHAD with GOD* class. The Scripture suddenly became alive and understandable. The Word is Spirit (John 6:63), she learned, which gives life to the teachings. Awakened from a spiritual slumber, Lili craved the pure, solid food spiritual diet (1 Corinthians 3:1-3; Hebrews 5:12-14; 1 Peter 2:2). Each session was like a drink of living water poured into her parched soul. Each subject was the Truth of the Kingdom of God revealed as never before. Out of the dusty pages of her Bible, Jesus Christ became tangibly alive. The new level of spiritual awakening juxtaposed her past of shame and guilt against Jesus' holiness and purity, a contrast between two worlds that can no longer be reconciled. Lili chose the best. Seated at the feet of Jesus, she heard the call to be transformed into His likeness (2 Corinthians 3:18), and she began to pray fervently for this to become reality in her life.

Lili was always connected to the religious observances of the Catholic Church. She recalled the memories of her mother praying the rosary, but she also recalled memories of her family engaging in occult practices. She admired her aunt, watching her skillfully form a circle of lit candles on the floor, reciting prayers, casting spells, and offering drinks to the attendees. She was well-known in the community as a shaman. Lili's young mind adopted a similar approach to spirituality, blending Christianity with occult practices.

A significant part of her childhood also included the many mysterious events, unnaturally appearing, tightly woven into her family's history. Most of them were a threat to her life, but each time, miraculously, she escaped the assault and even death.

Right from the beginning, just a newborn baby, she was found under the bed, crying. Everyone believed that a supernatural power threw her under the bed, because she couldn't yet roll over to fall or crawl to position herself under the bed.

As a very young child, she could see shadowy figures lurking in the dark hallways of her house, coming into her room. The images terrified her, especially the figure of a large dog, but there was no dog in the house. The encounters instilled deep fear, gripping her innocent soul with terror.

On one occasion, as a teenager, she played the Ouija board game with her high school friends in her room. Inexplicably, that same night, the room caught fire. Lili narrowly escaped. Undeterred, she continued experimenting with tarot cards, psychic readers, and Catemaco, Veracruz stones, wearing them as jewelry.

When in college, she continued to play the Ouija board game for fun. Unaware of the spiritual consequences, she shrugged off the warning signs as unwarranted coincidences. It was not until .... one beautiful morning, the coincidence was too obvious to ignore. As was her routine, with the Bible open on the table, she lit a candle, said her rosary prayers, and moved on with her daily chores around the house. A few minutes later, she noticed smoke coming from the prayer room—the Bible was on fire! Was it luck or was it a miracle, but the Bible was barely burned. The cover was slightly scorched, with no visual damage to the pages. Yet, Lili saw the Bible engulfed in flames.

As a young adult, Lili pursued true love only to experience painful betrayal. Her life was a mess of good intentions and bad outcomes. She felt trapped, abandoned, unwanted. Depression began to settle with no signs of an end to her misery. Her only strength came from her daughter, the delight in her life. Her presence defused the emotional fog she often found herself engulfed in.

Lili never connected her dreadful supernatural experiences to the occult rituals until, in the EHAD with GOD class, she learned of the biblical warning forbidding such practices. Oh, how sincere her repentance was! From today's perspective, she knew she had opened a gate for the enemy to take a foothold (Ephesians 4:27) in her life. The *EHAD with GOD* approach identified this area of her life as an impediment to her relationship with God. It had to be closed, and the enemy that was harassing her expelled.

After her penitence, Lili's spiritual encounters took a new height. The enemy became bolder in his pursuit to destroy her, but so was God in His pursuit to lovingly protect her. A new spiritual war unfolded, and Lili's soul was the winner's "trophy". The enemy was not hiding anymore, lurking in the dark. He threw at Lili every possible machination of circumstances, lies and deception, seduction and distraction, intending to destroy her mentally, emotionally, and physically. The marriage suffered the most. Her husband became unusually angry, verbally abusive, and on a few occasions, even physically assaulted her. This was not the man she married. His usual demeanor, being a quiet, almost timid man, had now turned into an aggressive and abusive monster. The more Lili grew into the image of Christ, the further her husband distanced himself from her, mistreating her badly. So did his family, throwing lies, accusations, assaults, and even wanted her out of his life. Lili was alone against a rapidly growing tidal wave of evil.

"This kind does not go out except by prayer and fasting," Lili remembered Jesus' words from the Scripture (Matthew 17:21; Mark 9:29). On her knees, Lili doubled down on prayer and fasting, seeking God's strength and guidance. She became action-resolute and family-committed, standing by her man. In the face of opposition and the risk of rejection, Lili was determined to do what was right in God's sight. She recognized the schemes of the enemy, called them out one by one, and cast them away from her family. She engaged in the war for her life, fighting for her loved ones. She ran into the daily battles head-on, ready to face the anticipated danger they presented. The *EHAD with GOD* clothed her with the Armor of God.

In the course of a year, Lili's heart was a battlefield; the frontline veered between defense and offense, wearing her down. Days of high confidence followed days of discouragement and depression. The emotional roller coaster drained Lili, her confidence wearing thin and confusion settling in—a despondency bordering on despair. Lili continued the fight with fasting and prayer.

Then, God spoke and the heavens decreed a time of favor. A series of dreams began to guide her through a maze of spiritual battles. Lili learned to distinguish between the dreams of the flesh from the dreams of God. She learned to recognize God's voice. At the time of each dream, she didn't have the complete picture, but as a sequence of events, they began revealing the spiritual reality behind Lili's encounters.

The first dream was a warning God sent long prior to Lili's enrollment in the *EHAD with GOD* class, much earlier before the troubles with her husband and his family began to unfold. In that dream, Lili saw herself outside of a house, rebuking the Devil. Many people were present, having a good time. They were talking between themselves, completely unaware of the despondent darkness that engulfed them. Being a stranger among strangers gave her the boldness to continue rebuking the dark presence. She paced herself through the rooms, holding a Bible and praying aloud. It was 3 AM when Lili woke up; her mind was still voicing the prayers from the dream.

"What was that?" Lili wondered. She didn't recognize the house, nor did she recognize any of the people in the dream. The next day was the day her Bible spontaneously burst into flames. Years later, when her husband brought her to his family's house, the sight took her by surprise. It was the house from this first dream. "What does God want to tell me?" Lili wondered. At that time, her prayer life was based on a routine, rather than on a relationship with the living God. How could she go around rebuking the Devil? Her prayers were more fearful than authoritative. She didn't read the Bible; as a matter of fact, she didn't even own a Bible after the fire scorched the old one. Lili kept all this in her heart with firm expectations that God, in the fullness of time, would reveal the mystery. And she patiently waited.

The second dream was preceded by a series of unfortunate events. Financial stress settled on the family. Her husband lost his job. She had a few opportunities to recruit new clients for her business, but somehow, all fell apart, and the potentials never materialized. Her husband became increasingly frustrated with her. He would lose patience with her and become very mean for no reason. They began growing apart. Lili recognized the attacks of the enemy and decided to play worship music in the house. She would sing along, and soon the songs would turn into prayers of thanksgiving and praise.

One night, as Lili was lying in her bed, an image of a man following her in the house ran through her mind. She tried to ignore him, knowing it was the enemy, but he cornered her.

"Do you want to listen to my music?" The man asked, but Lili ignored him. Another man approached her and spoke to her, his voice very irritated.

"Didn't you hear what the other said?" He asked.

"No! I don't want to listen to your music! Leave me alone!" Lili responded with a surprisingly firm voice. The pursuit continued, and so did she in her unrelenting indifference. She didn't want to engage the enemy. "If I ignore him, he will leave me alone," Lili reasoned. When it all ended, the clock glared at her with the 3 AM time.

The attacks on Lili's life intensified. Lili's mind became a minefield where old transgressions, forgiven sins, and redeemed practices exploded with guilt and shame. Voices incessantly claimed that her sins were unforgivable, that her daughter would be consumed with hate towards her, and that salvation was unachievable. The mental torture was augmented by physical symptoms. On one occasion, when bathing, the enemy appeared again, attacking her mind. Thoughts of worthlessness and statements of self-condemnation smeared her. The attack was so severe that she experienced a full-blown panic episode. A paralysis gripped her, unable either to speak or to move in her defense. At one point, she was not sure she could make it alive from the encounter. This assault crossed the spiritual barrier, causing her bodily harm.

The following two dreams were a two-day sequel, delivering one message. In the first, Lili was in an unknown house with her daughter; also present were many unknown people. This was kind of a gathering. People were talking, drinking, and having a good time. She found herself in a second-floor bathroom, and when she turned the faucet on, a very murky, unclean water poured out. The filth collected in the sink and clogged the drain. The carcasses of dead animals were floating in the water. The stench was horrific.

The second dream started where the previous dream ended. Again in the same bathroom, she turned towards the window, and the image terrified her: A huge tsunami wave, a giant wall of water, was rolling with great speed towards the house. The water color of the tsunami matched the water color from the sink. Mud and mire were coming at her, and there was no escape from the impending disaster. There was no time to get downstairs and find her daughter. Lili only had time to scream the name of Jesus. Slumped on the floor, she closed her eyes in anticipation of a violent end. The crash never materialized. The rest of the crowd seemed to be utterly unaware of the unfolding danger.

It was 3 AM hour when Lili woke up, both times, with a pounding heart. It was not hard for Lili to understand the meaning of the message because the same mud and mire were thrown at her in her real life. Soon after, her husband got arrested for spousal violence. His unwarranted hatred and the resentment toward Lili escalated in an ugly way, resulting in domestic abuse charges. His arrest was a new blow to Lili and the family. The spiritual war was claiming its victims.

Soon after the arrest, the enemy appeared again in Lili's dream. She recognized the man immediately. Their encounters had a history by now. This time, he dared to come to her own house, on her turf, to her family. His dark silhouette was outlined against the light damask of the living room couch, arms and legs widely spread as he lounged, taking most of the space. When he saw Lili approaching, the smirk on his face expanded in "delight." He began to taunt her.

"Remember me? You invited me long ago. I am just claiming what is mine. Remember the Ouija board? That was me."

"You must leave!" Lili spoke, surprised by the strength in her voice. The surprise widened when, instead of the terror from the previous dreams, she was filled with indignation, fueling her with righteous anger.

"Leave my house, now!" Lili repeated, her voice picking up strength with each command.

The man laughed and proceeded to speak again, but Lili's voice drowned his words with a steady stream of prayer.

"Jesus rebuke you, Satan. You are to leave this place and never return! This is my house. I claim this territory for the Kingdom of God! We are God's people. Leave, in Jesus' name!"

The man didn't budge. In a bold gesture to expand his presence, he spread his limbs, demonstratively claiming control over the house and the command of what happens within its walls. Like a rising stench from the pit of hell, the rising of his defiance and arrogance was palpable.

"Jesus, why is he not obeying?" Lili was bewildered by the ineffectiveness of her prayers. Instead of shrinking back in fear, she moved closer, standing her ground. From this position, she was now looking down on the man still sitting on the couch, asserting her dominance. The man found this boldness entertaining and dismissively gestured at Lili's efforts to intimidate him. His deep laugh bounced against the walls, and the echo carried the horrific sound throughout the house.

Lili lifted her arms to heaven, the only place she knew her help resided.

"Jesus, help me!" She cried, a desperate prayer for desperate times.

Help arrived immediately. The words were still on her lips when a transformation began to take place. A giant flashing sword appeared in Lili's raised arms. With its tip pointing down, she gripped the handle tightly. A power beyond her natural strength was given to her, an embodiment of "Christ in you, the hope of glory" (Colossians 1:27). With a supernatural might and a commanding voice, Lili drew the sword through the wooden floors.

"Be gone, Satan!" She shouted.

The impact opened a gaping hole; the abyss itself appeared, spewing fumes and flames under her feet. With a spiraling force, an invisible power sucked the man into the blaze, annihilating him within the eternal void of nothingness.

For a long moment, Lili stood speechless. The chasm below closed as it had opened in the blinking of an eye. The man was gone, and the right order of things was restored. And then, Lili saw it! Fitting perfectly over her delicate frame was body armor; she was clothed with the Armor of God! Tightly woven iron links formed a metal fabric that outlined her arms, tights, and chest. With a breastplate in place, she was girded for the battle. Lili woke up. It was 3 AM. Lili ran to the living room. The out-of-this-world scenes from the dream were in stark contrast with the peaceful settings.

"He is gone! The enemy is expelled!" Lili spoke to herself. A sigh of relief escaped her lips.

"Lord, you did it! What I couldn't do in the natural, you, my Lord Jesus, did for me in the spiritual realm. You fought the battle for me. You allowed me to witness all and be part of the victory. Thank you, my Lord!" Gratitude sprang from deep within her heart. Words of praise and prayer for thanksgiving filled the space. The presence of the Lord was tangible.

In the quiet of the early morning hour, the voice of the Lord rose assuringly,

"I will never leave you, nor forsake you" (Joshua 1:5; 1 Chronicles 28:20; Hebrews 13:5). "I no longer call you servant; I call you friend because I made the Father business known to you (John 15:15). You have been given to know the deep things of God."

This was a mountain-top experience. A place where heaven and earth meet, a new frontier where the spiritual and physical realms intersect. A new demarcation line was drawn, expanding the boundaries of the Kingdom of God on earth. The implications had eternal significance. The transfiguration of time and space into a delight and bliss resembled eternity.

"God fights my battles! He is my shield and protector. Blessed be your name, Jesus!" Lili prayed. The sweetness of the shared love could only be experienced, never described. And Lili was granted this privilege.

Life opened up with unexpected blessings. Lili got so much work that she had to look for a helper. Her daughter's private school reduced the tuition in exchange for some work on campus. The legal problems of her husband didn't go away, but the experience humbled him; he came to his senses, in contrition and penance. The humbled man she knew returned. So did the peace at home.

Lili became a devout believer. In prayer and worship, she served the Lord with gladness. Her love for Jesus reciprocated His love for her. The attacks of the enemy subsided, but she remained vigilant. Despite the assurance from the extraordinary events she experienced, she remained fearful that the troubles would return. That fear began gnawing at her peace. She even dreaded being in her house.

A new dream delivered unusual comfort. It was an entirely different dream from all the previous dreams. She didn't know, as the Apostle Paul said, whether this was an in-body or out-of-body experience. There were convincing circumstances pointing toward her soul leaving the body. One day, when united with the Lord, she would know the truth, but as for now, she knew that "The secret things belong to God, but the things revealed belong to us and our children" (Deuteronomy 29:29).

In her dream, Lili was taken to heaven. She saw inexplicable things and heard inexplicable sounds. But most of all, she found herself in Jesus' embrace. Floating in the midst of a diffused light, they remained embraced for a long time. Words of assurance and love were poured onto her soul. The worries vanished, and the fear was sucked out to be replaced by heavenly peace. The strong, yet gentle arms of Jesus conveyed love and protection. She leaned onto them, savoring the moment. Who would imagine that a mortal would be given such an honor—a divine embraced by Jesus while still walking the treacherous earth?

The WORD of God —The Weapon of War

Spiritual warfare is a war with prayer. The Word of God is our weapon. We don't fight against flesh and blood, but against the rulers, against the authorities, against the powers of this dark world, and against the spiritual forces of evil in the heavenly realms (Ephesians 6:12). When coupled with fasting, the power of prayer grows exponentially. If you have ever engaged in the occult, prayer and fasting are a must because these kinds of demons do not go away except by prayer and fasting (Mark 9:29). Demolish the enemy with these powerful words. Be on the offense! Memorize them, pray them as often as needed. Pray them before the enemy strikes. Pray them when you are in a battle; pray them even more fervently when you are at peace.

The prayer is structured on your identity in Christ, God's love, your power and authority in the spiritual realm, and true repentance and renunciation of wrongdoing. These are your fiery darts. The solidifying bond is Word of God. When prayed in faith, it reaches its target and accomplishes what it was prayed for. God takes no pleasure in the one who shrinks back in fear (Hebrews 10:38). Fight the good fight (1 Timothy 6:12) with the Word of God! Be victorious!

Prayer

I stand here today and confirm once again my eternal covenant with Lord Jesus Christ. I pray these words in His holy presence. May these words of my mouth and this meditation of my heart be pleasing in your sight, my Lord, my Rock and my Redeemer (Psalms 19:14). I declare them truthful and powerful. I put on the full armor of God, and I take my stand against the enemy of my soul, the Devil (Ephesians 6:10). Get behind me, Satan (Matthew 16:23, Mark 8:33).

I declare that I am a child of God. I am born again by the power of the Holy Spirit. I am a citizen of the Kingdom of God. I declare Christ as my inheritance. He is my life, my strength, my wisdom, and my beauty (Isaiah 61:3). My name is written in the Book of Life (Revelation 3:5; Philippians 4:3).

I praise the Lord because I am fearfully and wonderfully made (Psalms 139:13-16). Before I was formed in my mother's womb, God already had a plan for me. I am not a mistake (Psalms 139:13-16).

I claim the righteousness of Jesus through His finished work on the Cross (2 Corinthians 5:21; Romans 3:21-26). I am a planting of the Lord for the display of His splendor (Isaiah 61:3). Jesus has granted me authority and power to decree and declare, to bind and to loose, to bless and to curse (Matthew 16:19; 18:18), to trample on snakes and scorpions (Luke 10:19). I am called by the name of the Lord, and the enemy fears me (Isaiah 43:1-7; Acts 8:14-17). I decree that I am clothed in the power of the Lord. All who rise against me will be defeated before me. They will come at me from one direction and will flee from me in seven. I am the head and never the tail. God has blessed my lips and the work of my hands (Deuteronomy 28). Praise be to the Lord my Rock, who trains my hands for war, my fingers for battle (Psalms 144:1). Satan and you, demonic powers, you must obey when I speak to you.

The anointing of the Lord is upon me. I can do all things through Christ Jesus, who gives me the strength (Philippians 4:13). Greater is He who lives in me than he who lives in the world (1 John 4:4). My body is the temple of the living God, the living Spirit of God lives in me (1 Corinthians 3:16; 6:19).

God loves me (John 3:16). Satan, you cannot destroy our unbreakable bond of love (Psalms 18:1; Psalms 116:1). For I am sure that neither death nor life, nor angels nor rulers, nor things present nor things to come, nor powers, nor height nor depth, nor anything else in all creation, will be able to separate me from the love of God in Christ Jesus my Lord (Romans 8:38,39).

Satan, the finished work of Jesus Christ on the Cross has defeated and destroyed you. I claim victory over your darkness and speak the light of Christ over me. I speak life into eternity over me. I renounce and reject any agreement I have ever made with you, Satan, consciously or not. I reject and nullify any curses spoken over my life. I break any assignments against me. I speak confusion into the enemy's camp; let them destroy each other (2 Chronicles

20:22-23; Judges 7:19-23). I claim the blood of Jesus spilled on the cross for cleansing and protection. Be gone from my life! I cast you at the depth of the sea to never return to harass me again. No weapon formed against me shall prosper (Isaiah 54:17). Every demonic tongue that speaks against my life, let it be condemned. By the power vested in me by my Lord Jesus Christ, I break any satanic fiery darts shot at me. I break and cancel any satanic rituals, powers, assignments, and decrees against me, never to materialize in this world or in the world to come. Far from me, Satan! I belong to Jesus!

Angelic forces, I call upon you to come and assist me in my battles with the satanic hordes. Watch over my coming in and going out. Be by my side when I lie down and rise up. Be my hedge of protection (Job 1:10). Grant me safety from evil wherever I go. Guard my soul from defilement. Alert me to the danger of deception.

I release God's blessings over my family and me. I have the mind of Christ (1 Corinthians 2:16). May long life, joy, love, and prosperity be mine, in Jesus' Name. I declare these words of mine to have eternal prophetic power. They are reality on earth as they are really in Heaven. Today, I raise my Ebenezer as a sign of my victory in Christ (1 Samuel 7:12). I pray these words of declaration in the powerful name of Jesus. Amen!

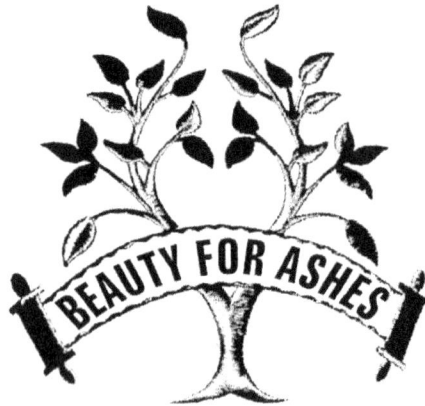

CONCLUSION

Salvation and Sanctification—Recap

How do I attain God's divine "raham/agape" love? The text below is a compact version of the *EHAD with GOD* methodology that leads the reader through salvation, sanctification, and ultimate transformation in the image of Christ Jesus.

Upon salvation, we are given **peace** (shalom) (Isaiah 66:12,13). As we progress through sanctification, we are endowed with **love** (agape). It is the spring of living water within, constantly overflowing for the benefit of others (Isaiah 12:3; John 4:13). Peace (shalom) is the state of inner tranquility of mind and heart. We are granted peace because of God's unconditional love for us. We acquire agape love when our love for God surpasses our love for ourselves. Peace and agape love cannot be contained within; they are a testimony to the transformation God has wrought in a believer's heart. The prophet Jeremiah testifies to this new reality, exclaiming,

His word is in my heart like a fire, a fire shut up in my bones. I am weary of holding it in; indeed, I cannot. (Jeremiah 20:9)

The believer's transformation also testifies to the overflow of what the heart is full of (Luke 6:45), namely, peace and agape love.

SALVATION—Peace Like a River

1. **BELIEF** in Jesus as Lord, God, and Savior for the remission of sin
2. **ACKNOWLEDGE** sin
3. **CONFESS**—verbal to a priest/pastor or inward prayer of confession to our high priest, Jesus
4. **REPENT**—Reject the sinful practices of the flesh and sincerely commit to removing them

Upon completing the above conditions, a person is JUSTIFIED and declared SAVED.

Prayer for Salvation

Lord Jesus, your Word says, "Everyone who calls on the name of the Lord will be saved" (Acts 2:22). I am now calling to you, Lord. I stand before you, Jesus, and humbly confess my sins and ask for your forgiveness. Forgive me for the sins I have committed against you and anyone, knowingly or unknowingly. Please come into my heart as my Lord, God, and Savior, and cleanse me from all my sins. I surrender to your kingship, and in faith, I entrust my life into your hands.

Lord, your Word says in Romans 10:9-10, "If you declare with your mouth, 'Jesus is Lord' and believe in your heart that God raised him from the dead, you will be saved. For it is with your heart that you believe and are justified, and it is with your mouth that you profess your faith and are saved." I believe, Lord. Your Word is Truth. Please grant me your salvation. May the Spirit of the living God come upon me and empower me to live a good life.

Grant me, Lord Jesus, victory over the sinful practices of my flesh by the power of your Holy Spirit. Thank you for saving me and for answering my prayer. In Jesus' name. Amen.

The key to entering the Kingdom of God is repentance. This is salvation. The key to remaining in the Kingdom of God is the practice of daily repentance and death on the cross. This is sanctification.

SANCTIFICATION—Love Like a Spring of Living Water

The commitment to become more and more like Jesus is to be transformed from "glory to glory" into His likeness (2 Corinthians 3:18). This is the willful process to empty myself from all that is mine (the practices of the flesh) and fill myself with all that is His (godly character). It is the daily acknowledgment of the deeds of the flesh (wrongdoing/sin) and the honest desire to get rid of their practices.

1. **CONFESS**—my daily wrongdoing/sin

2. **REPENT**—my daily wrongdoing/sin

3. **CRUCIFY**—my wrongdoing/sin—envision yourself putting your old self on Jesus' cross and driving nails through the sinful practices of the flesh, condemning them to death. For example, nail the anger, hatred, bitterness, judgmental attitudes of heart, unforgiveness, fear, addictions, gossip, etc., on the cross of Jesus.

4. **WASH IN THE BLOOD**—cleansing from the defilement of daily wrongdoings

5. **FILL UP WITH THE HOLY SPIRIT**—this is the seal of God that marks a believer for eternity.

Steps one through four constitute the **consecration** of the believer. It is the believer's conscious effort to cleanse themselves. Step five is the **sanctification** of the believer. Only God sanctifies and makes a person holy. There is no sanctification without consecration.

As a result of the above-mentioned steps, believers are set free from the practices of the flesh and no longer "crave" these sinful inclinations and desires. These practices have no power over them because their spiritual structures have been demolished; they have been subjected to death on the cross.

Prayer for Sanctification

Jesus, I confess my inability to conquer this sin _____ in my life. I now wholeheartedly repent of it. Forgive me, Jesus, for I have sinned against you. I now renounce this practice of the flesh and desire to turn away from it. I say "no" to it. I don't want this sin in my life. I hate it because it is evil. Lord, I now consciously exercise my free will to nail this sin on your cross. I desire to die to this part of my sinful, carnal nature. I declare this sin dead, and I turn away from it.

I call upon the cleansing power of Your blood to wash me pure from the defilement of this sin. Wash my mind and purify my thoughts. Wash my heart and purify its attitudes. Wash my mind, body, soul, and spirit, and make me whiter than snow, purer than gold, and shinier than the sun. Cleanse me, Oh Lord, for I desire to approach you pure in mind, body, soul, and spirit.

I now call upon Your Holy Spirit to come and gently fall on me. Come, Holy Spirit, and wash over, engulf, enter, fill, and sanctify. Heal the brokenness inside. Bring the healing of the Kingdom of God and restore me in righteousness and goodness as designed from the beginning of time. Restore to me the joy of Your salvation. Penetrate deep into my heart and my mind, sanctify me, and make Your dwelling within me. Teach me how to live a life of purity in the fallen and corrupt world. Guide my walk in the way to the Kingdom of God. Equip me with strength from above to resist the temptations of the Evil One, the world, and my flesh.

Jesus, I desire to be set apart for You. Holy Savior, make me holy because You are holy. Replace the practices of my old flesh with Your righteousness. Impart in me more of Your goodness, love, and peace. May Your righteousness be my righteousness and Your goodness, my goodness. May the life I live in this body be consecrated into life with You. May I no longer live, but You live through me. Amen!

NOTE: You may feel overwhelmed by negative emotions and find it difficult to forgive or even more, to love the person who hurt you. Your emotions might be so intense that they overshadow your rational thinking. While you may understand the importance of forgiveness, you might still struggle with feelings of vengeance and hatred. Here are some practical suggestions to help you navigate this difficult process:

GO WITH THE MOTION, NOT WITH THE EMOTION

Go with the motion of the cross, described in session one, using the prayers provided. Be honest, genuinely desiring to do what is right in the eyes of God. Don't trust emotions. The heart is deceitful above all things and beyond cure (Jeremiah 17:9). Instead, employ the strategy of simple faith: "The righteous will live by faith" (Habakkuk 2:4). Be completely confident that Scripture is truthful and the teachings lead to divine healing. Soon, you will be free from the burden of unforgiveness, and more importantly, you will find your heart yielding compassion toward your perpetrator. This compassion does not come from you; it is Christ's compassion for the perpetrator, since Christ lives within you. This is a manifestation of agape love and a sign of being EHAD with Jesus. You have been sanctified. You have overcome the enemy's schemes through the cross of Jesus by faith, not by emotions. You have met the righteous requirement of God's Law by loving your neighbor, even your enemies.

The Sacrament of Eucharist

The giving of the New Testament Covenant mirrors the pattern of the Old Testament Covenant. The ancient Israelites stood at the foot of Mount Sinai and made a covenant with God to follow and obey the Commandments He gave them through Moses (Exodus 20:1-17). God made the covenant with that generation and everyone born after them (Deuteronomy 29:13-14). Similarly, the sacrament of Eucharist is central to the New Covenant. The night before Jesus was arrested, He gave instructions on how to eat the bread and drink the cup in remembrance of Him. This covenant, like the one before it, was extended to all future generations yet to be born.

> This cup is the new covenant in my blood, which is poured
> out for you. (Luke 22:20)

The Old Testament covenant was sealed with the blood of sacrificed animals, sprinkled half on the altar and half on the people.

> Then he sent young Israelite men, and they offered burnt offerings and sacrificed young bulls as fellowship offerings to the LORD. Moses took half of the blood and put it in bowls, and the other half he splashed against the altar. Then he took the Book of the Covenant and read it to the people. They responded, "We will do everything the LORD has said; we will obey." Moses then took the blood, sprinkled it on the people, and said, "This is the blood of the covenant that the LORD has made with you in accordance with all these words." (Exodus 24:5-8)

The blood of Jesus spilled on the cross sealed the New Covenant. Jesus was the sacrificial lamb whose blood was sprinkled to cover the sins of the entire world, for those who were present and for all future generations yet to be born.

On Mount Sinai, a communal meal followed the giving of the covenant (Exodus 24:11). The Last Supper of Jesus and His disciples followed the same ancient pattern.

> While they were eating, Jesus took bread, gave thanks and broke it, and gave it to his disciples, saying, "Take and eat; this is my body." Then he took the cup, gave thanks and offered it to them, saying, "Drink from it, all of you. This is my blood of the covenant, which is poured out for many for the forgiveness of sins." (Matthew 26:26-28)

The Eucharist is the sacrament of the Church that renews the New Covenant, commemorating the sacrifice of Jesus on the cross each time it is celebrated. Jesus is the final and perfect sacrifice, sufficient to satisfy the just requirements of the Law of God, once and for all. As the perfect Lamb of God, His sacrifice has redeemed all the sins of the world that will ever be committed. Ironically, since the destruction of the Second Temple, the system of animal sacrifice has ceased to exist. For nearly two millennia, the blood of Jesus continues to supersede the blood of sacrificial animals. This fulfills the "new thing" that Prophet Isaiah prophesied about (Isaiah 43:19).

The "new thing" refers to God's New Covenant, through which He gives believers a new heart and places a new Spirit within them. He removes the heart of stone and replaces it with a heart of flesh (Ezekiel 36:26). The entire world benefits from this transformation, with the only condition being the acceptance of Jesus' sacrifice by faith. In commemorating His work on the cross, believers share the Eucharistic meal. The time of God's favor is now (Isaiah 61:2). When one accepts Jesus' sacrifice, they are saved, and their eternal destiny is changed from hell to heaven.

The ancient Israelites became indignant when Jesus said to them,

> I tell you the truth: unless you eat the flesh of the Son of Man and drink his blood, you have no life in you. (John 6:53)

Jesus referred to the spiritual meaning of the Eucharist, during which we partake in "eating His flesh" and "drinking His blood" in remembrance of His sacrifice—the price He paid for our freedom. The Eucharist is the highest expression of becoming EHAD with God: It is God in you and you in God (John 14:20). All who have accepted Jesus' sacrificial gift bear witness to the transformative power of the new life in Him that saves and heals.

There are conditions for taking the Eucharist. Apostle Paul passed to the believers the instructions he received from the Lord.

> Therefore, whoever eats the bread or drinks the cup of the Lord in an unworthy manner will be guilty of sinning against the body and blood of the Lord. A man ought to examine himself before eating the bread and drinks from the cup. For anyone who eat and drink without recognizing the body of the Lord eat and drink judgment on himself. That is why many among you are weak and sick, and a number of you have fallen asleep. (1 Corinthians 11:27-30)

We must examine ourselves! We are to examine our thoughts and actions, our attitudes and secret desires, as well as our relationships with others and with the Lord. If we neglect this self-examination, we risk falling under judgment, which can lead to various afflictions, including sickness and even death (1 Corinthians 11:32). The curriculum of *EHAD with GOD,* the entire journey on the narrow road you have undertaken for the last nine weeks, constitutes the act of self-examination. You have repented, rejected, and crucified the sinful practices of the flesh. You are cleansed in His blood and filled with His Holy Spirit. You have made yourself ready to partake in the Eucharist without fearing judgment. This self-examination must precede every Eucharistic meal.

Eucharist Prayer (after examination)

Lord Jesus, I have examined and found myself not lacking in standing to participate in your holy Eucharist. In faith, I take the bread and the wine, honoring your work on the Cross. With sincere gratitude, I commemorate your death and resurrection. It is life to me. I take the bread—your body broken for me—and I claim that You are in me, and I am in You, and we are EHAD. I take the cup—your blood spilled for me on the cross—and I claim that You are in me, and I am in you, and we are EHAD. Amen!

The Eucharist is the believer's mountaintop of transfiguration, where we meet with our Lord Christ Jesus in transparent holiness and purity. When taken without judgment, the Eucharist embodies the promised EHAD with God —God in you, the hope of Glory (Colossians 1:27).

My Agape Love Story With Jesus

Task: Reflect on your relationship with Jesus. How has your love for your Savior grown during your healing journey? On a scale of 1 to 10, how would you rate your love for Him before and after the *EHAD with GOD* course? (1 represents no relationship, and 10 represents a close relationship). Please compare your current ratings with those you provided on pages 43, 44.

Before

1	2	3	4	5	6	7	8	9	10
○	○	○	○	○	○	○	○	○	○

After

1	2	3	4	5	6	7	8	9	10
○	○	○	○	○	○	○	○	○	○

At the beginning of this journey, if you have given yourself ten (10), you have probably realized by now that you could not have loved Jesus with the same measure He loves you. We can't love on an agape level; we don't have the capacity to exhibit divine, unconditional love. However, as you sanctified yourself, shedding your old nature, you also shed (as part of your old nature) your own ability to love Jesus. The sanctification you have undertaken infused you with Jesus' peace and divine agape love. If Jesus were to ask you now, "Do you agape me?" what would your answer be? Agape oder phileo?

_____

_____

_____

Task: Self-love is paramount to achieving healing from trauma. What does your journey look like as of today? Please rate your self-love on a scale from 1 to 10 and discuss the reasons for this rating.

Love Myself

1   2   3   4   5   6   7   8   9   10

◯ ◯ ◯ ◯ ◯ ◯ ◯ ◯ ◯ ◯

Discuss your thoughts

_____

_____

_____

_____

_____

_____

_____

_____

_____

_____

_____

EHAD with GOD

REFLECTION—Week Ten

Reflection 1: Confidence in God's healing—before and after scores

Reflection 2: Reflect on your "Give Him Five" time praying to Jesus

Reflection 3: Daily confession and repentance in prayer to Christ—our high priest; crucify the flesh, wash with the blood, fill with the Holy Spirit (page 13)

Reflection 4: Well-being Scale for self-evaluation—before and after scores

Task: Reflect on your "Give Him Five" time praying to Jesus. How did the practice of His presence evolve? See page 41 for a comparison of before and after. What changed?

_____
_____
_____
_____
_____
_____
_____
_____
_____
_____
_____
_____
_____
_____
_____
_____
_____
_____

Well-Being Scale For Self-Evaluation

Date _____

Evaluate four areas of your life affected by traumatic events. Mark your responses with "X" to the question: "How am I doing today?"

HOW AM I DOING TODAY	GREAT	NOT SO GOOD	BAD	REALLY BAD	MISERABLE
PHYSICALLY					
EMOTIONALLY					
SPIRITUALLY					
RELATIONALLY					

Physically—My overall health. How solid is my night sleep? My appetite, chronic conditions, current diagnosis, and quality of everyday life.

Emotionally—Volatility of feelings, ups and downs of emotions, bouts of anger, rage, depression, manias, panic attacks, hatred, etc.

Spiritually—Relationship with Christ, ability to worship corporately, read the Bible, personal prayer time, assurance of salvation, sense of God's presence.

Relationally—Quality of familial relationships and circles of friends.

Task: Compare your initial results under session one, page 47. Notice any changes in your functioning in the four areas of life before and after? Discuss your findings.

_____
_____
_____
_____
_____
_____
_____

Encouragement and Follow-up Instructions

You have endured in faith through challenging teachings, lengthy counseling sessions, and powerful prayers for your sanctification and transformation in the image of Christ. You have not only learned, but you implemented these teachings in your life. By sanctifying and transforming yourself in the image of Christ, you have taken a critical step toward your healing. As it is written, "The kingdom of God is not a matter of talk but of power" (1 Corinthians 4:20). Through this power, you set yourself free from unredemptive emotional pain and misery. I praise the Lord for the treasures He has stored in you through your healing.

Even though the instructions end, my involvement in your healing does not. Send questions or inquiries directly to:

shaynah@thetraumahub.org

Shout your testimony of freedom from the rooftops. May the Lord God, our Father, honor your effort by freeing you from the bondage of emotional pain and misery forever.

> Guard the good deposit that was entrusted to you—guard it with the help of the Holy Spirit who lives in us. (2 Timothy 1:14)
>
> Only let us live up to what we have already attained. (Philippians 3:16)
>
> May the God of peace sanctify you through and through. May your whole spirit, soul, and body be kept blameless at the coming of our Lord Jesus Christ. (1 Thessalonians 5:23)

Amen!

APPENDIX 1, 2

PHYSICAL TRIAGE

Cancer	Bone Disease
Allergies	Muscle Disease
Sinus Problems	Female Reproductive System
High Blood Pressure	Lung Disease
Arthritis	Kidney Disease
Heart Disease	Ulcers
Diabetes	Brain Injuries
Liver Disease	STDs/AIDS
Migraine Headaches	Thyroid Deficiency

MENTAL HEALTH TRIAGE

Health Issues	**Health Issues**
Anxiety Disorder	Suicidal Ideations
Bipolar Disorder	Schizophrenia
PTSD	HDAD
Depression Disorder	Panic Attack
Substance Abuse Disorder	Autism
Eating Disorder	Personality Disorder

SPIRITUAL TRIAGE—FEAR

Fright	Performance
Torment	Fear of Being Judged by Others
Nightmares	Fear of Poverty
Fear of Death	Fear of Dark, Heights
Timidity	Claustrophobia
Shyness	Fear of Abandonment
Inferiority	Fear of Pain
Inadequacy	Fear of Men (due to past abuse)
Rejection	Fear of Authority
Worry	Fear of Evil Spirits
Tensions	Fear of Parental Authority
Stress	Fear of Failure

PRACTICE OF DIVINATION

Mediums	Spirit Channeling
Horoscopes	Tarot Cards
Satanism	Palm Readers
Mutterer (talking to oneself as with a spirit)	Games (Dungeons and Dragons)
Witchcraft	Crystal Gazing

Astrology	Mysticism
Ouija Boards	Transcendental Meditation
Spiritual seances	Fortune Tellers
White Witchcraft	Eastern Religions
Santeria	Voodoo
Gothic Music/Clothing	Wicca Practice
Ashram Pole Worship	Other

SEXUAL ASSAULT

Molestation (child)	Sex Trafficked
Molestation (adult)	Rape
Incest	Sold into Prostitution

SPIRITUAL STRONGHOLD (BONDAGES)

Rationalization of the Word of God	Blasphemy
Unbelief	Atheism
False teachings	Defilement
Irritability when Reading the Bible	Loneliness
Irritability when in Church Services	Hopelessness
Resentment	Bitterness

Contempt	Anger
Envy	Shame
Pride	Laziness
Control	Gossip
Coveting	Greed
Jealousy	Gluttony
Alcohol	Idleness
Pornography	Hatred
Debauchery	Lust
Adultery	Fornication
Immorality	Falsehood/Hypocrisy
Deception	Stealing
Fame	Money
Mistreating Parents	Arrogance
Lying Tongue	Lack of Trust in God
Drug	Judgmental Attitude
Disrespect for Authority	Sexual Misconduct
Self-pity	Spiritual Slumber
Shrinking Back from Life	Doubt

www.ingramcontent.com/pod-product-compliance
Lightning Source LLC
Chambersburg PA
CBHW081357270326
41930CB00015B/3326